GW01606361

DON'T BLAME THE BRAIN

The Missing Link Between Emotions & Inner Peace

JULIA PAPPAS, M.ED/CAGS, NSCP, CPC

Copyright © 2023 by Julia Pappas

All rights reserved. No part of this book may be reproduced, stored, or distributed in any form or by any means without the written permission from the author, in accordance with copyright laws.

Needs-Based Emotional Regulation Process (NBER Process™) is a trademark of Julia Pappas. Unauthorized use is prohibited and is subject to all applicable laws.

Limits of Liability and Disclaimer of Warranty: The contents of this book are provided for general informational and educational purposes only. Neither the author nor the publisher can be held liable for the use of the information provided.

Library of Congress Cataloging-In-Publication Data

Names: Pappas, Julia

Title: Don't blame the brain: the missing link between emotions and inner peace / Julia Pappas, M.Ed/CAGS, CPC

Identifiers: LCCN 2023907038 | ISBN: 9798218188061 (paperback) | ISBN: 9798988293507 (hardcover) | ISBN: 9798988293514 (ebook)

LC record available at https://lccn.loc.gov/2023907038

Cover design: Darko Dojcinovski
www.behance.net/DareDD & darko.dojcinovski@gmail.com
Interior illustrations: Courtesy of the author

DON'T BLAME THE BRAIN

The Missing Link Between Emotions & Inner Peace

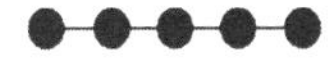

JULIA PAPPAS, M.ED/CAGS, NSCP, CPC

To all those seeking

to connect with their sense of

vitality and aliveness

Contents

Author's Note

This book is a resource. As with all resources, it may help you a lot or a little. Everything depends on your unique situation and your needs. Although the tools offered in this book may be life changing for you in a positive way, I am also counting on you to think for yourself and decide what applies to you and what doesn't. I hope that you will take what works for you and leave the rest, but also realize when you may need someone else by your side to walk you through difficult emotional experiences. And finally, information offered in this book is in no way intended to replace clinical management, formal counseling or therapy, as well as pharmacological treatment, for those who need it.

Introduction: Why This Book

Does the world really need another book on emotions? Don't we all have several of them on our bookshelves?

Yes and yes.

Yes, we have many books on emotions. Too many perhaps. My own shelves are buckling under the weight of all the books on emotions that are in my collection. From emotional intelligence to emotional regulation and processing, there is no shortage of books, it seems. And yet, we do need another book.

Not one more book.

But *another* book.

A different kind of book.

The kind of book that actually gets you *excited* about emotions. Perhaps even looking forward to them, wanting to feel more and feel deeper.

So why do we have so many books about emotions and why do we need another one? Firstly, because emotions are inseparable from us. They follow us around and we follow them. They can cause a lot of distress and discomfort if we don't know what to do with our emotions or why we have them, and so we all want answers.

Understanding and processing emotions is key to how we feel at any point in the day and how well we function overall.

The second reason (which, in my opinion, is the most important) is — *getting it right*. It's important to get it right when we process what we feel. We cannot run away from our emotions, cannot hide from them, and cannot tell ourselves we don't feel what we feel. At least not without a huge cost to the quality of our lives. So when we don't do it *the right way*, we end up carrying double the burden — the unresolved and misunderstood emotions themselves, but also the burden that comes from avoiding or denying them.

So fine, you may say, aren't there books out there that tell us exactly how to do it right?

There are a lot of books that attempt that. But most of them miss one critical piece, and that makes them *almost right,* but not quite. It's like a great dish that is missing a pinch of salt to bring out the true flavor. Having studied innumerous publications in professional literature and having read multiple popular books on the topic, I can see that almost all of them are missing the point. Let me explain.

When it comes to dealing with emotions, what is the most common advice? What do you often hear?

In one way or another, most books say something like:

- *"Your thoughts cause your feelings"*
- *"Change your thoughts in order to feel better"*
- *"Retrain your irrational brain"*
- *"Sit with emotions, watch them come and go"*

Chances are, you've been trying to do one or more of these things. Well, let me ask you... Is it working? Has it really worked for you and *how well*? How hard do *you have to work* in order to see any results? At the end of the day, don't you feel like there is still something missing? I certainly do. Not only have I seen these recommendations flop in my own life (and I am a skilled psychologist, so that certainly sucked), but they failed all the time for my clients (which sucked even more!) as they tried but struggled to truly make progress with these outdated methods. And so now, when we work together, we do something completely different.

After years of observations, critical thinking, personal reflections, and some creativity in my professional work — *I finally realized how to articulate what the missing piece was.* You see, thoughts do not cause feelings. And there is nothing wrong with your brain. This should not come as a surprise to you. Deep down, you knew this to be true all along. The evidence for that can be seen in our failed attempts to trick our brain or to change our thoughts in order to feel better. It doesn't work because we are focusing on the wrong thing. Emotions are not caused by thoughts and they are not triggered by "outdated programming" in the brain either. They come from *another* place. Yes we think about emotions, but our thoughts don't cause them.

So, what does?

And what do we do with our emotions?

Glad you asked!

That's what this book is about and I cannot wait to give you the answers. I am sure you are as hungry to know as I was when I was looking for the missing link between strong emotions and inner peace.

Before we begin, here is something I want you to know. I never intended to write a book. I would much prefer to read one instead! But my clients insisted. They craved a different way of processing emotions and found my method very effective. They also wanted to have it in a written form, to refer back to and to share with others. The funny thing was, my method seemed so common sense to me that I was sure it had been written about already. And so I went looking for a book that would have the same answer I gave my clients on how to move from emotional distress to feeling at peace.

Unfortunately, I couldn't find that book. I tried. After searching for several years, I decided that even if a book that describes my approach is out there somewhere, the fact that it has been so hard to find, meant I had to write it. And so I did.

The method I am about to teach you has the missing link that most books don't talk about. This method will make processing your emotions so much easier! I wish someone had just told me this simple thing that I came to learn through my own discovery, personal life experiences, and countless sessions with clients (both adults and children). I wish I had this book earlier in my life to learn from and to share with others. I am so happy it's here.

Enjoy this book and feel good, finally!

Chapter 1

Why Do We Still Struggle With Emotions?

I could start this book with a chapter about the brain. I could tell you what the brain does to shape our perception of emotions, the role of neurotransmitters, and so on. It would be grounded in scientific theory and, perhaps, even look impressive. But because I've found information like that not to be really helpful or practical for people I work with, I won't waste your time either.

My hunch is, you'd skip the brainy chapter anyway to get straight to the heart of the matter. So why don't we skip it together and get to the practical things right away? Besides, we don't really have to discuss neurons, synapses, and neurotransmitters. Why? Because emotions have more to do with your *whole being as a human*, as opposed to one organ in the body, the brain.

While I don't think neuroscience and brain chemistry are what we need for context in order to move forward with our conversation, what may be helpful is to understand some of the reasons why emotions still present such a challenge (despite all of the available theories). And no, it isn't because we need more brain research. So let's begin with a question:

Would life be easier without emotions?

Although a spontaneous answer may be — yes, if you take a pause and think about it, you'd probably be reluctant to part with *all* of your emotions. You'd probably want to keep those feelings of peace, bliss, joy, ease, etc.

Everyone seems to like positive feelings.

So then, would life be better without the *negative* emotions? Isn't it the negative emotions that make life unpleasant? We may be tempted to believe so. There are certainly many books suggesting that not only is it possible to live without the whole spectrum of your emotions, but that this is what we *should* strive for. I wholeheartedly disagree with this idea. And I hope you will disagree with it too, long before we reach the end of our conversation.

You see, it isn't the negative emotions that make our lives difficult. It's *what we do* with them. You may be surprised to hear that emotions are actually meant to make life easier, not harder. We just need to know what they are for and how to use them.

As you will soon see, emotions are the most sophisticated and intelligent thing we have as human beings. Speaking of intelligence, what's commonly understood by the term "emotional intelligence" is often confused with *social intelligence*. And it is also usually reduced to the ability to use "appropriate" labels for your emotions (i.e., how precisely you can name an emotion), the ability to perceive emotions in others, and the ability to accurately describe and express your emotions to them.

However, the true key to emotional intelligence is the *ability to know what to do with your feelings* in a particular situation and *how to resolve them* successfully. And when I say "resolve" I do mean making a negative emotion go away, as opposed to simply managing it or making it tolerable. And guess what? In order to do that, you don't need to know the precise name for that feeling nor do you need proper words to express it to others. The way I see it, you can use a screwdriver even if you don't know it is called a screwdriver. You just need to know what it's for. Same with emotions.

Like all good tools, emotions have a purpose.

You can benefit from them tremendously if you understand what to do with them. Once you grasp one simple principle behind your emotions, you will be on your way towards living a much better life. The kind of life that isn't possible if emotions are either ignored and suppressed or, at best, simply tolerated. I hope that you will be able to reach the point where not only you embrace your emotions, but also come to have a deep appreciation for them and the work they do on your behalf.

It is understandable, however, why we might think life would be easier without them.

Truth be told, emotions can present quite a challenge and we often do find ourselves at a loss for what to do when anger, anxiety, or hurt rise up within us. So let's explore some of the reasons why we still struggle with these feelings. Answering this question would be helpful in terms of giving us some context for where we will go next in this book, but it may also offer you insight into why you personally may be finding emotional experiences not so easy to deal with.

But first, let me tell you a personal story of how I got here.

MY PROFESSIONAL DILEMMA

There is a plethora of tools and strategies when it comes to dealing with emotions. Sounds like a good thing, right? Yet, this is the main reason so many of us still struggle. You would think that, for someone like me, having formal training in the field of mental health would be a great advantage when it comes to processing emotions. You get to learn *all* of the tools. Awesome, right? Uhm, not quite...

Though my training did help with things like holding supportive space for others, labeling emotions, building communication skills, helping people with conflict resolution, de-escalating triggering experiences, and so much more, when it came to the actual tools of *working with emotions* — a lot was left to be desired. This wasn't for the lack of variety in the tools offered, but rather because of my ongoing skepticism about the effectiveness of those tools and strategies in bringing about long-lasting outcomes.

I was introduced to various methods for dealing with emotions. From cognitive-behavioral models to mindfulness to biofeedback, you name it. Some of them were interesting and promising, others — quite dry. As you may suspect, studying theories is one thing, but applying them in real life — that's another story. Real life is the real test. What I found was that the more formal the framework was, the more dull it sounded, and so it was less likely that my clients would buy into it. And why would they, if I didn't either...

But why was I so skeptical?

First of all, I do not like the idea of *buying into* something. I don't like it when I have to believe something will work, in order for it to work. I don't want to rely on the placebo effect. I want things to work, regardless of what I believe about them. Can you relate? Emotions may be nebulous, but the way we go about them doesn't have to be fluffy or impractical.

But there was another reason I was skeptical. You see, prior to my formal training, I already had my way of processing emotions. I had an understanding of where they came from and what to do with them. It was very different from what I was taught, but it was intuitive and worked just fine.

Everything new I was learning throughout college and grad school was naturally compared and contrasted with what was already working for me. Although I did have to learn these models (because they were considered to be "the best practice" in the field), they felt too clumsy to be relevant in my own life. And so I sat in my classes, I studied the textbooks, I wrote long papers, and I passed my exams. I earned my degrees with excellence and distinction. But other than that, I moved on with my life and continued to use my own way of processing emotions.

All was good, until I started working with clients and tried applying the models I was taught in my practice. I figured, even though those methods aren't useful for me personally, they may work for others. Why else would they become the "standards of practice"? I quickly found that, besides a temporary relief, the results they offered were never quite satisfying or long-lasting, but rather superficial. They *seemed* to work because we really *wanted* them to work. The belief they will work was required. The placebo effect was strong.

But even the placebo has its limits. This temporary relief was only achievable around lighter feelings, as opposed to resolving heavier emotional distress.

Something was off.

No matter how hard I tried to teach my clients the standard ways of thinking about their emotions, I wasn't feeling it any more than they did. Clearly, it wasn't working. Not only was it ineffective, it also wasn't the thing I was doing personally in order to resolve difficult or uncomfortable feelings of my own. And so I started wondering... Why am I teaching people to do the things I myself don't find particularly helpful? Why teach tools I do not personally use? The answer my mind gave me was that I was doing *what I was taught to do*. But what my heart was telling me instead was to do *what I know works*.

Best practices aside, what guides our professional practice as psychologists and mental health professionals is our code of ethics, which urges us to put our clients first, ahead of any models and tools. No matter how commonplace or fancy they may be, if the tools don't work, we don't blame our clients. We change what we do. And so, armed with this conviction, I gave myself permission to follow my heart and put those "brainy" frameworks from my training back on the shelf.

I couldn't believe we were doing things backwards, and I couldn't believe how long I tried to make these things work for others. I kept thinking: why contort ourselves into ridiculous positions of the mind in order to change our thoughts about how we feel? Why use gimmicks and tricks? So instead of teaching my clients how to "believe new thoughts" or how to "outsmart their brains" out of feelings, I showed them my process.

And it worked.

Why wouldn't it?

It worked for me all the time.

It dawned on me then that I should have made the switch much sooner. Not only does this process work, it is also *so simple*! And the simplicity isn't even the best part. The best part is that emotions do feel resolved in a *genuine way*. The kind of way that tells you there is something profoundly natural about it. As one of my clients said: "I feel like I don't have to lie to myself anymore. This is so simple. I don't have to overthink my feelings. It just clicks."

Ever had the feeling of something being "just right" because it feels so effortless and natural, like it is supposed to be that way? That's exactly what I am talking about. Perhaps the best analogy for this would be like trying to fit a puzzle piece into a section of the puzzle where it *looks like* it's the right piece. It seems like a good fit because of its color and shape and it *sort of fits* into the gap... Except, it doesn't slide in there effortlessly.

As much as you'd like this to be the piece for that section, your fingertips can tell — it simply isn't. You may try again and again to jam that piece in there, to make it work, but deep down you know that if it isn't sliding in place on its own, it doesn't belong there.

That is how I've been feeling about the models, the methods, and all the tools available out there — like I was trying too hard to make them work, and that the real answer was elsewhere. And once I realized what the answer was, when I found the missing link to emotional regulation, quite literally — everything clicked into place. Like it was always meant to be there.

I cannot wait to share that missing link with you.

In this book, I will show you the process that I follow and teach others, so you can try it on for yourself. But before we do that, let's first consider why, after so much research and so much literature on the subject, do we still struggle with emotions?

HERE IS WHY WE STRUGGLE

The reason why we struggle with emotions is because we've been *doing it wrong*. We either overcomplicate them or, on the contrary, we downplay their importance. When the importance of emotions is downplayed, we don't feel validated in what we feel, and so we end up resenting our feelings. Even if we don't resent them and do try to understand what is going on, we may place too much emphasis on the wrong things — such as naming and describing them (for example, what color or shape our emotions resonate with). We might use other ineffective tools or try to express feelings to other people in hopes that they will know what to do with them. And in the end, we settle for a temporary relief, not realizing that there are better answers.

Does any of this sound familiar? That is why we still struggle with emotions. Let's look into each of these reasons in more detail. And I hope that you will be able to see that there is *nothing wrong with you*, but rather, the issue lies with the tools we've been offered.

1. Over-complicating emotions

The first reason for why we still struggle with emotions is that we overcomplicate them. For something so basic and inherent to our human nature as emotions, one would think that understanding them should be pretty straightforward. And perhaps it was, until we turned it into a matter of scientific investigation.

As it often happens in academia, the language surrounding the topics under study becomes more and more complex in order to support various theoretical frameworks. That in turn makes that language and the frameworks it describes inaccessible for day-to-day living. This tendency is quite evident in brain research, which is flooded with inaccessible terminology.

Perhaps, if the matter was atypical and so highly specialized as, let's say, seizures, then having experts talk to experts in "expert speak" makes sense. But for the frequency with which each one of us has emotional experiences, easy to understand "no-brainer" solutions are a must. I am not saying we don't need brain research or that perhaps, at some point, there may not be useful insights from it. There may well be. What I am saying, however, is that we cannot put our lives on hold waiting for some magic answer to come out of laboratories.

Typically, results from most studies are often inconclusive, require corroboration, and have little practical application out-the-gate. So while these studies continue, instead of holding our breath, we should go on with our lives and use methods that already work.

It falls to practitioners in the field, like myself, to decipher relevant research and make it useful. Still, even then, things don't appear to be less complicated. When it comes to books and articles on emotions, lectures and talks available to the wide audience online, there is still this tendency to get overly technical. Yes, there certainly is a difference between moods, emotions, affect, and feelings, but guess what? This distinction is not that relevant when we want to know what to do with what we feel. Not to mention that the plethora of terms is likely to make us feel inadequate and dumb.

Since these technicalities do not truly assist us in understanding what is going on with our internal world and do not improve your experience as a human being, we will not dwell on them here. Labeling the sensation you get as a feeling or as an emotion does not change how you need to approach it. There is no need to further complicate a process that has been made unnecessarily confusing already.

As you will see in this book, emotions are not at all confusing.

It is the labels and the terminology employed that make it so. So for the sake of simplicity, we will use the words *emotion*, *feeling*, and *mood* interchangeably to refer to an experience of emotion (i.e., to anything you feel).

2. Downplaying the importance of emotions

The second reason why we still struggle with emotions is the flip side to the first one. This is where we may over-simplify and dismiss what we feel to the point of nullifying any significance it has. I believe this comes from a misunderstanding of emotions and their purpose (something we discuss in the next chapter). This happens when we try to convince ourselves that emotions are a somewhat annoying and useless remnant of human evolution. How many times have you heard that "reptilian structures" in our brain are the reason for our emotions? And how many times have you seen the advice to not listen to the "lizard brain"?

However unimportant we may try to make them, it doesn't change the fact that emotions keep showing up on a regular basis. They *keep making themselves important* by the manner of their impact on our day, our ability to pursue goals, and complete tasks. If something has that kind of power of impact, it simply is unwise to dismiss it.

Not talking about the elephant in the room doesn't make the elephant go away. Having an elephant in the room may be awkward, but not talking about it — makes it ten times worse. However, that's exactly what we often do with our emotions — we treat them like the elephant in the room. I mean, who would want to admit that they let their "reptilian brain" control them? No one. If we believe that emotions come from a lesser and evolutionarily inferior part of ourselves, it makes sense why we would want to suppress them. The good news — we don't have to. Emotions have nothing to do with the "lizard brain," a concept we will revisit in Chapter 9, so for now let's leave these poor animals alone.

No matter how much we are being told that emotions are not relevant to modern humans, it does not change the fact that we *do have* them and *do feel* their impact, quite a significant one at times. When we hear that emotions are not that significant, we may feel stigmatized by our inability to squash them down. We may be wondering what's wrong with us, why can't we ignore them and rise up above "the limbic system" (another debated scientific term) into the "higher mind" (what does that even mean?). I find these terms confusing and unhelpful, and yet they appear everywhere.

These types of terms drive us to pathologize normal feelings, making us believe this is something we should have outgrown, and that having them makes us less mature or advanced. This erroneous assumption as to the utility of emotions in modern life comes from a deep misunderstanding of the fact that triggers and threats in modern societies are *just as real and vital* to our survival as they were to our ancestors. Sure, we may not be fighting with chimps over bananas and territory and may no longer be living in caves, but we do still want our own place in the sun, as they say. We do have to be vigilant on the road while driving, provide for our families, and avoid dark alleys at night. It's life, it just looks different.

3. Resenting our emotions

The third reason for why we still struggle with emotions is that we begin to resent them. Naturally, if we are exposed to either of the two previously discussed ideas — that our emotions are just too complex to be understood or just too irrelevant to be bothered with — we will eventually feel helpless and resent having them.

How does it feel to live with something you resent, something you cannot walk away from, or find constantly irritating? Horrible, right? Definitely does not make for a good relationship with ourselves and it leads to a constant internal battle.

Instead of being validated in our experience every time we have an emotion, we think that something's wrong *with us.* We blame it on feelings and start believing that life would be easier without them. We tell ourselves it is all in our head, that events in our lives are neutral, and that our worries are made up in our minds by false beliefs and automatic thought patterns. In doing so we fall victims to our own gaslighting. In other words, we manipulate ourselves into believing a reality that deep down does not feel real. And what does that accomplish? It feeds the vicious cycle of resentment: the more we tell ourselves that it is all in our head or that it is all because of how we think (as opposed to something truly not being right), the more invalidated we feel.

The more emphasis we put on the thinking part and the more we tell ourselves that emotions are caused by thoughts, the farther away we move from the true answer. Remember that puzzle piece analogy I mentioned earlier? Well, it is kind of the same here, where we want that piece to fit in so badly that we are willing to hold our finger on it at all times to make sure it stays in place. Which does beg the question of whether it truly belongs there, doesn't it? Because the minute we let go, that piece pops out. No matter how much we tell ourselves that our thoughts are causing our feelings and no matter how hard we try to control how we think, it does not take care of that nagging feeling that something is inherently wrong with that approach.

The feeling of resentment is a very strong and negative one. Resenting emotions, out of all things, further amplifies the negative experience. If we do not know what to do, we will avoid dealing with resentment, just like we avoid dealing with any other negative feeling. We avoid looking at resentment, just like we avoid the people we resent. But just like in relationships, no matter how much we avoid facing it, we cannot get away from it. Avoidance does not resolve resentment, whether we are talking about emotions or people. And as our resentment persists, so does our struggle with emotions.

4. Emphasizing naming and description

Since resentment doesn't lead us anywhere, eventually we may decide to try something new. So instead of avoiding feelings altogether, we do the opposite — we zoom-in on our feelings and start paying attention. And I mean, *real close* attention. We are told to be very specific about what an emotional sensation is like. Does it have a temperature? What color is it? What shape? We are told to spend as much time as needed naming and describing it, until that emotion goes away.

We think that maybe if we can name it, we can "tame it." And if we can see it, we can "free it." And if we can tap it, we can "zap it." Although it may sound fun at first, this is yet another reason why we still struggle with emotions. Why? Because even though we may be paying more attention here, we are paying attention to *the wrong things*, like the color of emotion, its location in our body, its shape, size, and other imagined qualities.

What does that do?

It shifts our attention from feeling *to thinking*.

And it is not a helpful type of thinking. It's the kind of thinking that is distracting us from the reason we have that emotion in the first place. So instead of wondering why that emotion is there and what we need to do about it, we focus on finding its proper name. Which one of the hundreds of emotions is it? That should take us a while! In assigning physical and sensorial attributes to our emotions that, let's be honest, have little to do with their true purpose, we are turning emotion processing into a cerebral task. This further strengthens our bias towards a cognitive "brainy" approach to feelings. In other words, it transforms a sensation into a set of sentences about it that have nothing to do with its true origin, its purpose, and its outcomes.

The best analogy I can think of to illustrate how unhelpful this is, is a burning flame. The flame will serve as a metaphor for emotion in this case. Let's say a house is on fire. That's quite concerning, right? We should do something about it, shouldn't we? But what if, instead of figuring out how it needs to be handled, we focused on describing it? How big are the flames, what particular color do they have, are they dense or light, are they spreading or seem contained, and on, and on. And what if we spent as much time as it takes doing only that until the flames burn out. Problem is, the flames may be gone, but so is the house. A similar story happens with our emotions. Meaning, even though they do eventually go away on their own, they leave us depleted, unresolved, and sometimes — burned out.

5. Relying on empathy from others

Relying on empathy from others is yet another reason for why we still struggle with emotions. Some people will tell you that the problem with emotions is that we do not express them enough. Ok, at first that sounds promising. Until you find out that by "expressing" emotions what is really meant is "expressing emotions *to others*," the premise being that emotions have social value and have to be communicated to other people.

In other words, we are being told that the value and purpose of emotions is social: "to communicate them to others." That is not so, as I will show you in this book.

According to this school of thought, the reason why we have trouble with emotions is because, as a society, we lack "expressive skills" to communicate and articulate our feelings to others. Because if we did, we would be able to relieve the burden of carrying an emotional experience alone. And so, they say, the answer to resolving emotions is to have more opportunities to express them to others. You may say, "Yeah, that sounds pretty good to me. What's the problem with that? Isn't it good to express an emotion to someone and let them know how you feel?"

Indeed, this may sound great if you have a particular someone to turn to every time you have an emotion. Especially, if that someone has the kind of skills necessary to assist you in getting to the root of your emotion and can help you understand what needs to be done about it. Truth is, not many people have these skills, and those that do are not always available. Yet emotions show up 24/7. Another reason why expressing an emotion to others may sound great, is when we look at it from the perspective of the one who is expressing it. But imagine returning the favor and being on the *receiving end* of someone's emotions. Would you feel as excited, and for how long?

Carrying other people's emotions for them would get tiring pretty fast, wouldn't it?

Compassion fatigue is the reason why most people will not be able to support us this way, just as we too wouldn't be able to offer ourselves like this to others. Not to mention, the level of responsibility that this puts on the shoulders of those who are asked to make space for our emotions, is unreasonable.

In holding other people responsible, it at the same time disempowers us. So not only does it imply that it is the other person's responsibility to understand and validate us, it also makes it their responsibility to help us process and resolve whatever that emotion is about. That's a big ask! And is not a fair one. No one should be tasked with our own work.

Of course, receiving empathy is a beautiful experience when we are struggling with emotions. Problem is — empathy is not a commodity and there isn't always a listening ear.

While we go around searching for empathy, we miss the opportunity to help ourselves sooner. The more we wait for someone else to support us, the more we continue to struggle. But if we know what to do, we can support ourselves independently and through any emotional experience. Some practice may be needed, of course, but it is absolutely doable. We can definitely be heard and seen, if we learn to hear and see ourselves. How do we do that? Through our emotions. (I know I didn't give you the answer yet as to *how to do that*. It does require a whole book, so please keep reading.)

6. Seeking relief over resolution

Another reason why we struggle with emotions is that we settle for *relief* over getting the real answers. This, of course, is understandable, since emotional experiences can be quite burdensome and we may not feel compelled to spend any more time feeling them and reflecting about them.

We may stop asking questions as soon as we feel some relief, because we believe that it is all that's available to us. And so we think that we'd better enjoy this moment of peace while it lasts, because we certainly know it's going to be brief before another negative feeling shows up. Given that the tools usually offered to us to help with emotional regulation often provide only temporary relief, it is natural to assume that all we have to do with discomfort caused by negative emotions is — to seek relief.

And so as soon as we feel a bit better, we move on, not realizing that there is more for us here. We are not aware that there are bigger truths and much more satisfying answers to our discomfort. Getting to these answers provides long-lasting and impactful resolutions.

Who would have thought that, instead of simply a relief, we could actually gain strength, confidence, reassurance, nurture, and even wisdom. What?! Is that even possible? Yes. If you go a step beyond simply being aware of your emotions, if you stop waiting for them to pass, and if you ask certain questions that we will get into in the chapters that follow, then — yes.

Even when I ask my colleagues about whether these models and processes (thought therapy, meditation, etc.) work for them, they all say that they work "to an extent" — which is precisely my experience. Some of them also add with a sigh something like: "...suffering is part of life and part of the human condition."

I sigh too, though not in agreement.

Lack of good tools can certainly make us believe that achieving what we want may not be possible. And it may not be, especially when we don't have what we need. But when it comes to emotions, I think we can do better than using models that only work "to an extent." And, I do not agree that emotional suffering is inevitable. Discomfort and tension may be inevitable. Complexity is there too, because humans are complex.

But do we really *have to suffer* due to our emotions?

Or, do we suffer because we don't know a better way?

I believe suffering from our emotions comes from not having access to the right tools, answers, and resources. And the good news is that all of this is available. It's time to put down what doesn't work and try something different. Before we do that, let's take a look at one more reason.

7. Blaming the brain

There are many more reasons why we struggle with emotions, and I could go on and on. But I will make this the last one for the sake of moving us closer to solutions. This reason is all about blaming it on the brain.

We do this a lot. And we hear others do this all the time. It has become the norm in the self-help industry. Basically, it is anything we say to ourselves and others that suggests that our brains are somehow "behind," have not kept up with evolution, are built wrong, or are malfunctioning. In other words, it is a brain-problem that we are confused about emotions, cannot think straight, don't know what we want, or how to get there.

But is it? If it is a brain problem, then what do we do about it? How do we tangibly impact our brain? How do we change it? Noise, noise, noise! These are the wrong questions to ask. They are pointless. You cannot change something you do not have direct access to. And if you do have a sense that you've changed your brain, it is probably because it wasn't the brain you were working on to begin with. So, I invite you to ponder with me over this:

What is the point in blaming the brain?

It's just another organ in our body.

Is there anything we can practically do about the brain's anatomy and function? Can we direct when and how your neurotransmitters fire?

No. We don't have such control.

Although motivational pep-talks and stories in the mainstream media do promote the idea that "if only we could think differently, we would change our brain's chemistry," we can always use our own discernment. There is a big difference between *metaphors, theoretical hypotheses,* or even *promising findings* in science, and real tangible tools you can use right away. As of the time of this writing, we are not practically equipped to manipulate our brains and cannot monitor how our thoughts change our brain chemistry.

Taking the brain apart piece by piece and checking for "what's broken" is not something we can do. Not because we are missing the manual, but because there is none. And none is required. Your brain is not broken. We are not supposed to focus on the brain in isolation.

We are meant to look at *our being* as a whole.

If your brain is structurally healthy and you are not under the care of a neurologist, then your brain is not the problem. You see, the brain is an organ that helps orchestrate an action. But it is not responsible for *the reasons* behind the action or how it is executed, and so on. These are all the things that we evaluate through the lens of our mind, our own being, our consciousness, our attention and awareness. Pick the word that most resonates with you here.

The point is, it is *we* who decide what to do. The brain simply helps us get it all in motion. A car analogy may be helpful here. Although the car gets us where we want to go, it is us who decide where we are going, how fast, and whether we follow the rules of the road along the way.

If you are wondering why you are not getting what you want and you are blaming your brain for it, you found the wrong reason. The real reason why you are doing the wrong things or getting poor outcomes is not because of your brain. It's because of an insufficient level of understanding and intention behind your actions. And this is true for emotions as well, because in order to resolve them, we must take proper actions which depend on our understanding and awareness of how this process works.

The brain is not in charge of what is in your awareness. You are. Your consciousness is. To do better, you need to fine-tune your awareness and understanding of how to resolve emotions. That is when things change. We will talk a lot about awareness in this book. The whole model I am offering you is comprised of 3 Steps of Awareness — but we will do so in actionable and practical ways.

I hope this will lead to many positive changes in your life.

Let's begin.

Chapter 2

Your Thoughts Don't Cause Your Feelings

I mentioned in the previous chapter that emotions are meant to make our life easier. But in order to see how, we need to understand their purpose and why they occur. Where do emotions come from? Are they caused by our thoughts?

There are many myths out there about emotions and their purpose, but believing that emotions come from our thoughts is easily *the biggest* one of them all. And we need to start here first. It may be so ingrained in us that, unless we resolve it, it will get in the way of seeing a new perspective on where emotions truly come from.

I am not going to name names, but if I did, rest assured the names would include many of the people you know. From professors, to coaches, to motivational speakers, to media personalities, and so on. You've heard them speak, you've read their books. The biggest names in the fields of mental health and personal development are promoting this message in some variation or another.

It may sound something like this: *"Your thoughts create your feelings."*

- Or: *"To change how you feel, you need to change how you think."*
- Or: *"We don't react to circumstances, we react to our thoughts about them."*
- Or: *"If you don't like what you feel, choose better thoughts to think."*
- Or: *"We don't have negative emotions, we have negative thoughts."*

Or some other version of the same idea. The bottom line of what is being communicated here is that our brain imagines a problem where there is none. Basically, they say, our brain has a tendency to "make it all up." And it does that supposedly because it has an "outdated program" running in the background that is no longer relevant for our modern life. Like a software full of bugs, they say, it makes up thoughts about seemingly neutral things, which then create our unpleasant emotions. Something triggers thoughts in our brain, which then triggers emotions. Or so they say.

But how true is that, actually?

Not at all.

THE BIGGEST MISCONCEPTION

The notion that our thoughts cause our feelings, is not only popular, it is *assumed* to be correct. The number of books, treatment manuals, and research publications based on this notion, is quite impressive. So then, it *must be* true, right? The sheer volume of material promoting this idea should be enough to convince you to accept it as the normal way to think about this causal connection between thoughts and feelings.

But not so fast, I say.

To agree with this notion, that thoughts cause our feelings, we also have to agree that before humans had thoughts, they had no feelings. Because when we say that thoughts cause feelings, it is implied that thoughts come first, before the feelings. So — following this logic — until we were able to think, we were unable to generate feelings. In other words, per this claim, in order for someone to feel anything they must first be able to think. And not just think... One must think the kind of thoughts that trigger a particular feeling. And, if you are daring enough to take this claim even further, it would mean that unless someone has cognitive processes that can support conscious thought, that someone would have no experience of emotions.

Obviously neither is true.

We can easily prove that not only thoughts do not cause emotions, but that emotions are actually quite separate from thoughts and have a life of their own. (Ever had a feeling you had no words for, which means you also had no thoughts for? Then you know what I am getting at here.) Thoughts do play a role, but not the role of a trigger for emotions. More on that in a bit.

Before humans evolved to think and to communicate with words, emotions were already there, signaling to them about something important. You can also observe a young child who has no language, but clearly has a rich emotional life. And just in case you are thinking that a young child may not have language but has thoughts, which supposedly would support their rich emotional expression, let's consider a newborn in order to see how this isn't the case. A formal, organized, self-reflective thinking process is simply absent in an infant. Yet this is precisely the kind of process that is required in order to have *the power to cause* anything, let alone an emotion. What you see an infant do is spontaneous, immediate, and reflexive in its nature. Their brain is simply not developed enough to have thought processes that have direct causal connections to any other thoughts, or feelings, or actions.

And yet, even at this stage of development, an infant is capable of both positive and negative emotions and expresses them spontaneously and clearly. If you have been around infants, not only do you know they feel and express negative emotions with intensity (so as to make sure they are attended to), but you can also differentiate an angry cry from a sad one, both of which are distinct from a cry that arises from fear. Clearly, it isn't the thoughts of an infant that give rise to these feelings. This is the most direct evidence of emotions arising *without* thoughts. We do not need to have thoughts in order for emotions to arise.

But to make this point even more obvious, let me ask you this.

Have you been around dogs?

If so, I do not need to tell you that dogs also have feelings and display them too. And so do other complex mammals, by the way. You can certainly tell the difference between an angry bark and an excited one. Likewise, you can tell that a dog is angry, sad, or scared by the sounds it makes, its body language, etc. You see these signs because the dog is experiencing these emotions.

Now, let's answer this question. What triggers the dog's emotions? Do the dog's feelings arise from its thoughts? Do we tell the dog to change its thoughts in order to change how it feels? (And why would the dog "want" to change how it feels?) How about that baby? Should we solve its cries too by suggesting it works on his or her thinking?

That sounds pretty ridiculous, doesn't it?

Yet, somehow, we think that this is what *we* should do. Why? How did we get here? We will explore why in just a bit. But first I want to make sure we drive this point home — that *emotions exist outside of our thinking*. In other words, whether or not we think, we most definitely feel. Feelings can rise without a thought, and we can feel an emotion without a particular thought driving that emotion. In fact, what I want you to understand is that our emotions are not driven by our thinking, although we can certainly have thoughts *after the fact* and can certainly think *about* what we feel and why.

When it rains, you bring an umbrella with you.

But umbrellas don't cause rain.

And since our thoughts do not cause our feelings, it is naive and erroneous to assume that in order to change how we feel, we have to change what we think. A thought process is not required in order to feel an emotion, as we have seen in the case of an infant and, beyond that, in mammals as well. So if thoughts are not the cause for an emotion, attempting to change our thoughts may be completely irrelevant to what gave rise to that emotion to begin with. Therefore, changing thoughts may not be sufficient to change what we feel, not to mention that the tactic of changing thoughts may not even be possible (as in the case of a young child, for example).

THE PRE-VERBAL QUALITY OF EMOTIONS

The reason why emotions occur irrespective of our thoughts, is because they have *pre-verbal* quality. Prefix *pre-* means "*before*" and indicates that something occurs *prior* to something else. In case of emotions this means that they occur before, or prior to, the words that express and articulate our thoughts. Even if those thoughts are about a particular emotion, they do come *after* the emotion, and not before.

You can have thoughts *without emotions*. For example, when I think 5x5=25, I am not feeling anything about that thought. This is an example of a thought occurring without an emotion. Likewise, you can have emotions *without thoughts*. For example, we have an emotional and often spontaneous reaction to music, or when we suddenly catch a whiff of summer blooms, or when we are moved by a breathtaking view. These are examples of emotional reactions without a thought behind them. If we had to think about every experience that causes emotions in order to have that emotion, we would live a very disjointed and confusing life, not to mention we would miss out on many things. If I had to think about how beautiful the rose is or how wonderful its fragrance, *before* I enjoyed it, I would miss out on enjoying it until I properly thought about the qualities worth enjoying.

This simply does not make sense and, thankfully, that is not how it works. Like I said earlier, we may have thoughts *about* our emotions, but we don't need thoughts *in order to* have an emotion.

And just like we want to be able to enjoy things spontaneously, we also would want to be alert to potential problems just as quickly. This is why language and thoughts are not pre-requisites to having emotions. This pre-verbal quality allows them to occur without the barrier of language. And that should also help us understand why believing that emotions are caused by thoughts is not only unhelpful, but it isn't actually true at all. Look at the non-verbal or pre-verbal manifestations of emotions (e.g., in pre-verbal cultures of early humans, in babies, mammals, etc.), and you will see what I mean. The evidence of emotions stemming from something other than thoughts — is right there.

This pre-verbal quality is the very reason why we see emotions manifest so clearly in infants and pets. When a baby cries, you can tell an angry cry ("Feed me now") apart from a sad cry ("Play with me, I feel lonely") and a fearful cry ("Pick me up, I'm scared").

Although emotions are always about something, they are usually *not* about our thoughts. Babies and dogs, most definitely, are not having a thought process that leads them to feeling what they feel. And there is also no direct way to impact their experience with "alternative" thoughts. These are great examples of what I mean when I say that emotions are pre-verbal. Simply put, if it's not about words, words won't cause it and words won't fix it. Pre-verbal children, and even children who do have some command of language, don't have enough metacognitive skills to think about what's causing their frustration, or sadness, or worry. Not only that, they are incapable of causing those emotions *with* their thoughts. Children barely have the capacity to think, let alone think *about their thinking*, and yet they still feel a full range of basic emotions.

And when I say basic, this is not to imply they are primitive or underdeveloped.

Basic emotions means fundamental emotions.

We have such a big range of what we feel, with some emotions being loud and clear, while others — more subtle and nuanced. Yet what they all have in common is that they stem from only a couple of basic emotions. These basic emotions — happiness, anger, fear, and sadness — are the foundation of all other feelings. Another reason why they are called basic is that they are universal and reflect common human experiences. And not only are these emotions shared amongst all people, animals have them too.

Why is that?

Because emotions are essential to survival.

That is the meaning behind the word *basic* — they are essential.

They are so essential, in fact, that we never "outgrow" them (because we are not supposed to, but more on that later). They are part of our biology. That is why we see emotions arise in babies and dogs without requiring a formal thought process. Here are some important things to note about emotions:

- Basic emotions stay with us throughout our lives.
- They make it easy to understand how our life is going.
- They tell what, if anything, needs to change.

The fact that they are basic, makes them easy to understand in ourselves and others, even when they are expressed in a nuanced way. Just like we can tell the difference in various emotions in a baby, we can also tell that difference within ourselves. We too, have basic emotions that are core to our experiences and that, in some form or another, show up on a daily basis, depending on the particular "flavor" of the situations we are in. We may not know *what kind* of sad, or angry, or fearful we are feeling, but we definitely can tell them apart from one another. And if you are struggling even with that step, don't worry, I have a process for you to get you unstuck.

The point is: these basic emotions arise in response to the environment and without thinking, because of their pre-verbal quality. This pre-verbal quality is not accidental, nor is it a pitiful remnant of evolution. It has quite an important role and, as they say in the world of software development, *it's a feature not a bug*, which is to say that what may look like a flaw is actually intentionally designed to perform a certain function. What is that function in emotions? Let's explore.

AN EVOLUTIONARY FLAW?

Even though the mainstream message is that emotions are a flaw of evolution, quite the opposite is true. Emotions have a very vital role to play in our wellbeing, otherwise they would have been eliminated through evolutionary processes. Nature is not known for generating unnecessary complexity. Were they not *essential*, emotions would long be gone.

Considering how much energy they take and how much of our attention they demand, there must be something really important about them, don't you think? Not only have they survived all other evolutionary changes, their preverbal quality makes them that much more powerful and impactful. This is what helps emotions to *by-pass our conscious thinking processes* (which happens to be yet another argument against the idea that thoughts cause emotions) and rise to our awareness quickly. And for a good reason. This is to ensure that emotions are able to perform their function, with or without words and thoughts.

That function is — survival.

Emotions are vital to our survival and for that reason, whether we have words and organized thinking processes or not, emotions will show up to signal about something very important. So important, in fact, that the more we try to over-analyze and push thoughts ahead of our emotions, the more likely we are to miss the whole point of why they are there to begin with. The longer we continue believing that our thoughts are causing our feelings, the longer we will stay in the dark and struggle with our emotions. Because in trying to change our thoughts, not only are we *not* changing our emotions, we are missing the point of *why* emotions exist. And so what is the purpose of emotions?

Emotions exist to *ensure our wellbeing*.

This may sound counterintuitive at first. Especially when you consider the fact that we don't actually feel a sense of wellbeing when we experience anger, sadness, or worry. However, this will make more sense if we think about emotions as only signals, alerting us and making us aware that our wellbeing may be at stake. And so the cause of discomfort is not emotions themselves — nor is it our thoughts for that matter. Most definitely not. What is it then? It is the changes in our environment that compromise our sense of wellbeing in some way, which is then expressed through emotions. And so, it should make sense why a negative emotion signals some compromise to our wellbeing, whereas a positive emotion signals a restored sense of wellbeing.

If our general sense of wellbeing is compromised, our ability to live a balanced and fulfilling life is also compromised. Our wellbeing is closely connected to our survival and, therefore, needs to be monitored. Any threats — perceived or real — to our wellbeing need attending to. Our emotions make sure we pay attention to people, places, and things that threaten that sense of wellbeing. And so it would make sense then that, when something is critical to our survival, it would have an immediate and reflexive quality. Perhaps even appear impulsive, due to its instinctual nature. That is why sometimes emotions feel automatic and reactive, because — they are. Since their purpose is to communicate to us something important for our wellbeing, the way this communication is designed supports that function. It is immediate and direct, which also means that it bypasses conscious and intentional thinking.

This process is *the result* of our evolution, not an accident.

The signal in the form of emotion is direct and immediate on purpose — to ensure *we attend* to our wellbeing. So whereas, it is not our emotions' direct purpose to make us feel good, they do *prompt* us to do what needs to be done in order to maintain a sense of wellbeing. It is *our job* to respond to emotions in a manner that restores our sense of wellbeing. You know that to be true because you, just like me, take actions to feel better when you don't feel good about something. Sometimes we may not know what to do, but we always feel the urge for it.

As I'm showing you on this image, emotions increase our alertness and prompt us to scan our environment. During this scanning process, we think and reflect on what is happening and what is having an impact on us. It is from this scanning process, which we can also call "assessment," that we get a sense of what's impacting our wellbeing and can take action to restore it back to balance. It is a good thing to think about our emotions and where they came from (trigger), so we can better understand what to do about them (action).

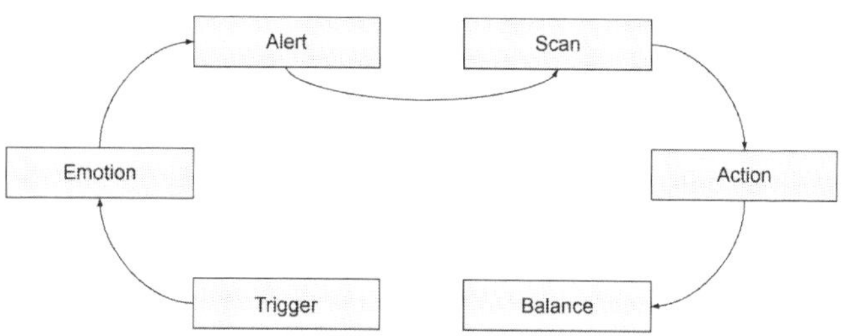

The problem is, of course, that we do not always do what's wise or what's in our own best interest. And if there ever was a flaw in the world of emotions, it is this — our own failure to respond to emotional signals in ways that most serve us (e.g., eating cookies after a stressful job assignment or binge watching a show after an argument with a partner). But that is a conversation for another chapter, which we will surely have.

One thing is certain — believing that emotions come from thoughts is not a wise way to respond to them. If, in response to a negative emotion, we try to change it by talking our way out of it and by manipulating our thoughts — we are doing ourselves a disservice. Why? Because in doing so, we are missing an opportunity to change something about the *actual* cause of discomfort. And since the cause is not the thoughts, we shouldn't be wasting our time trying to change them. So what is the cause, you may be wondering. Let's talk about that next.

WHAT TRIGGERS EMOTIONS?

If it's not our thoughts, *what then is the cause of emotions*?

Most of the time, emotions arise in response to a change in our surroundings. When something is not right, a negative emotion arises. A baby may be crying when left alone or when the diaper is dirty. It's uncomfortable, something doesn't feel right, and needs fixing. "Time to go to bed" is pure injustice in the eyes of a toddler, just like "no more video games" or "time for homework" is injustice from a teen's perspective. You can expect some strong negative reactions here in the form of anger or sadness.

None of these things feel great to those who experience them and they do threaten those individuals' sense of wellbeing. Who doesn't want to play and have fun? Why would anyone want to interrupt what's working great for them in place of something that, in their eyes, is either irrelevant (like sleep) or boring (like homework)? So of course, these events will result in strong emotional reactions (and protests), which serve to preserve and protect all the things that make one feel a sense of wellbeing. And by the way, your opinion as a parent in regards to the value of sleep and homework is, unfortunately, irrelevant.

In other words, our own understanding of what does and does not contribute to a sense of wellbeing is not going to change the significance of these experiences in the child's own eyes. What we deem important may not be what the child finds meaningful to them. Not to mention that *our thoughts* about their feelings will not change what *they feel* and why.

If you are having trouble connecting with a child's perspective and their experience here, let me illustrate a similar situation that involves an adult. Let's imagine you are enjoying a chat with a friend over the phone. Perhaps you haven't spoken to them in months and now is the time to catch up. Two minutes in and you get interrupted by your children who hurriedly tell you that the cat got inside the dishwasher and that, in trying to get it out, they accidentally closed the door on it. The point is, someone interrupted what you were so happily enjoying and messed it up for you with something "really important," which also happens to be the last thing you want to be dealing with.

How might you be feeling in this scenario?

Probably irritated. Perhaps frustrated or maybe even furious, if a similar cat situation has happened ten times already that morning and none of that was an accident. Now, we could try and pretend that it is your thoughts that are causing your feelings, and we could also attempt to change your thoughts in hopes that you would feel better. But let's be honest, you will not be on board with that. No matter what someone tells you, you feel what you feel because of what just happened *around you*, as opposed to inside your head. Other people's opinions about your feelings will not change your feelings. Ironically, this further supports the point that thoughts and opinions come *after emotions*, and that they alone will have little to do with changing these emotions. In fact, what will make you feel better is an action taken that corrects the problem and restores your ability to talk with your friend.

What you do and what actions you take depends on your particular situation (and how far out of control things may have gotten). Do you lock up the cat? Do you lock the dishwasher? Or do you lock up the children? Jokes aside, how you resolve the problem of interrupted phone calls depends on your assessment of that problem and what you see as available solutions. But one thing is clear, your actions most certainly would not be focused on you changing your thoughts and pretending like nothing happened.

Now, this is not to say that thoughts are irrelevant. Not at all. We don't want to dismiss our thoughts completely. They do have a role to play. But it is important to get the order right so that we understand what role thoughts play when it comes to emotions. They do play a role, just not the role of *causing* them. Our thoughts help us *process* emotions, they help us reflect on our emotional experience, they allow us to ask questions about the trigger, as well as help us find solutions. A solution is a proper action that restores our sense of balance and wellbeing.

Of course, we also cannot ignore the fact that we do have a lot of negative thoughts when we experience negative emotions. (We may be thinking things like: "Why is this happening?" or "This isn't fair" or "I don't deserve this...") The only difference is that these thoughts are not the *cause* of your emotion. They are a *reaction*. The *emotion* is the cause of your thoughts, *not the other way around*. Negative thoughts appear as your brain kicks into gear to note the feeling, try to analyze the situation, understand the problem, and figure out what actions need to be taken. All of this is well and good, except that if we are not aware that this is exactly what our mind is trying to do — however ineffectively sometimes — we create a problem by trying to shut down this thinking process. What we should do instead is engage in an active and intentional form of problem solving, and not in a coercive "thought correction" also known as "thoughtwork."

When something threatens our wellbeing (in ways big and small), that signal gets communicated immediately and it calls on us to pay attention. It is what we do with that attention and how we think about that signal (i.e., emotion), that matters most. That is where our thinking comes in, and in many ways seems to have led us astray. Not our emotions, but the way we think about them. Now, this is a subtle, but very important, difference. We can think about our emotions, but we do not cause them. And how we think about emotions may or may not be helpful.

Emotions trigger our thoughts.

As they should.

They are, in fact, designed to. This is the way they alert the brain to a potential problem. As shown on the diagram earlier in this chapter, emotions alert us and initiate a "scanning" process. They signal to the brain to examine what may be impacting our sense of wellbeing and also prompt it to look for solutions.

Too often we focus on the wrong "problem" — the emotion itself (because we make it to be the problem). However, emotions are nothing but a messenger that signals about a potential issue. They are not the problem itself. If we engage in various means of avoiding the messenger, we may eventually succeed in eliminating the signal, but not the actual issue that prompted this signal to begin with.

It is like deactivating a smoke detector. It may stop detecting the smoke and stop sounding the alarm when the smoke is there, but it won't make the smoke go away. Sure the sound of an alarm is very unpleasant and the idea that there is something wrong and needs to be attended to — may not be the thing you were looking forward to dealing with. And yet, if there is a problem, wouldn't you rather know about it than be oblivious to it? Wouldn't you want to know if there is smoke in your house, even if the sound of the smoke detector is highly unpleasant? Most certainly.

And one more point... We often think of emotions as *the cause* of the problem. And if we continue with the smoke detector analogy, then it is like saying that the smoke detector caused the smoke. Which is, obviously, not the case. It tells you the smoke already *is* and is *detectable*. Unless, of course, your smoke detector is malfunctioning, which is a separate story. We are working off of the assumption that everything is in a good working order and that you are a functional person with functional — though misunderstood — emotions.

So let's be clear about this sequence:

- Emotions arise *before* thoughts.
- Emotions *activate* thoughts about them.

This is the order, and not the other way around. Our thoughts do not cause our emotions. It is our emotions that cause our thoughts.

This is so *on purpose*. A signal in the form of a specific emotion reaches our awareness, so that we do something about it. In order to do something about it, we have to employ our thinking, because it is through our thinking and our assessment of the situation that we will understand what to do next. And so the emotion will rise to call attention to something, something worth paying attention to. The signal will be strong enough for us to notice it and think about it. And that is why emotions trigger thoughts on purpose, so that our thinking can direct an action that addresses whatever is the concern brought to our attention by that emotion.

INCONVENIENT, BUT NOT PROBLEMATIC

Emotions may be inconvenient, but they are never problematic. What do I mean by that? Consider this scenario... You are at work, and someone calls in with a message for you. If this is a personal message that is urgent and critical for you to know, would you prefer to be interrupted or would you rather it waits (until the next day or whenever you have time for it)? Of course you would want to receive it immediately.

Now, what kind of message rises to the level of urgency will depend entirely on our personal circumstances (for example, something happened to our child at school or our flight got canceled). However unimportant it may seem to someone else, if *we* deem something to be urgent and important, we would drop everything to attend to it.

Urgent messages like that may certainly be inconvenient. Normally we would prefer not to be interrupted. Yet, we would rather be interrupted for something we consider truly urgent and important, than to not be aware of it at all and end up missing it completely. In other words, even though urgent calls are inconvenient, they are not problematic, and we would rather they do get through to us.

You see, the same applies to emotions.

When they show up, and especially when they have a high intensity to them, they are urgent messages that require our attention. They do interrupt whatever we are engaged in. Although they may not be convenient and may show up when we least expect them, they are not problematic. It is our thinking and bias against them that makes our emotions to be the problem. We assume our life would be better without them. We would rather not have them, so that we don't have to deal with them

It is thoughts like this that cause trouble, not our emotions.

How we think about what we feel can get us in trouble.

Our ability to interpret our emotions, understand what they mean, what triggered them, and what to do about them is what dictates whether the way we process emotions is helpful to us or not. Essentially, if we do not understand *the trigger*, then *the action* we take may not restore *the balance* we want.

For example, if we have a problem with a coworker, would binging on ice cream solve that problem? It may certainly make us feel better because it is a fun distraction, but does it actually fully resolve the emotion? Next day when we run into the same frustrating issue at work, should we fix that frustration by eating even more ice cream? Or should we instead focus on the source of that frustration and decide how we may approach the issue with our coworker?

We have a choice. We could either *cover up* an emotion (by eating ice cream) or *resolve it* (by fixing the problem itself). If we cover it up, the problem will reoccur and will trigger the emotion once again, to prompt us to address the actual trigger. How we address the problem and resolve the trigger will depend on the nature of that situation. And so thinking about the trigger and understanding it — is key to finding proper action.

You see, it is not the emotions themselves, but how we think about them and what we decide to do that is either helpful or not. And a lot of the time, it is our thinking about emotions that is incorrect and problematic, as opposed to the emotions themselves. When we push emotions away, we ignore the trigger and miss the opportunity to resolve it.

We have talked about the reason behind our struggles with this in the previous chapter. The very idea that emotions are caused by thoughts, stops us from finding solutions and prevents us from attending to our wellbeing. When we think this way, we interpret emotions as false alarms, and focus on fixing our thoughts, which keeps us stuck in our heads even more. We miss the fact that emotions are pre-verbal and can not be triggered by our thoughts.

When you understand that emotions are vital to your wellbeing in a very specific and direct way, you will stop trying to change them. You will also stop resisting or ignoring them, and stop seeing them as problematic. Instead, you will want to attend to them, no matter when they come up or how inconvenient they may be. This is why the pre-verbal quality of emotions is so critical. It allows for the emotional transmission to go directly into our awareness, unobstructed by language, and send us a message.

But what is that message? Why is it urgent, and what is that vital and direct connection to our wellbeing? What is it about our emotions that, once they occur, makes it hard *not* to think about them?

The most important thing to understand, as we wrap up this chapter, is that emotions call to us *before* we are even able to think. Most of our thinking occurs *after* the emotion gets our attention. And the reason for that is because our emotions signal to us about our wellbeing and our needs. Understanding this is critical to resolving challenging emotions and restoring our sense of balance and wellbeing. That's what the next chapter is about.

Chapter 3

What You Really Need & 3 Steps To Get There

Earlier I said that we never "outgrow" our emotions. The notion of rising "above them" (as if our thoughts are somehow superior to our feelings) is based on the assumption that emotions are a nuisance. Outgrowing our emotions, trying hard to change them, or "getting over" them would be like getting over our most essential qualities. And since this goes against human nature, it is not going to happen. As we discussed in the previous chapter, basic emotions are called basic because they are essential to our wellbeing. Our capacity to have emotions is like a navigation device that points in the right direction.

That direction is our wellbeing.

So what you really need is to learn how to navigate.

Based on our earlier discussion, you now know that emotions are not caused by thoughts per se. Of course, when we think about an upsetting event, we will re-experience negative emotions associated with it. However, it is important to understand that it is still *the event itself*, rather than our thinking about it, that is causing an emotion. For example, your boss was extremely rude to you. That's upsetting. Days later you are still thinking about it and feel upset. You are not upset because of your thoughts about it, but rather because it is an upsetting incident, no matter when you think about it. And until the incident is resolved through an appropriate action, it will continue to be upsetting. We cannot "correct" our emotions by simply thinking differently about what happened or by searching for positive thoughts about an otherwise upsetting event.

But then *what do you do* and exactly *how* do you process emotions? And if it isn't our thoughts that we have to change in order to feel better, then what is it? These are the questions we will answer in this chapter, and I already left you a hint (which is — taking appropriate action).

"WHAT'S WRONG WITH YOU?"

If you are not happy with how emotions show up in your life or how little things seem to trigger reactions you don't want, you probably said to yourself something like: "What's wrong with you?" If you had tried any of the things that didn't work, you also might have thought that there is probably something wrong *with you*, because these things "should" work. I can relate.

Something *is* wrong.

But not with *you*.

When we have no answers and when emotions feel trapped inside of us, it is hard not to blame ourselves. But I hope to give you a completely different approach in this book, so that there is no need for that. And before we move on to Step One: Emotion Awareness, here is what I want you to do.

Reflect along with me...

If you are a parent, think about what your child does when they are sad, angry, or scared? If you are not a parent, think about yourself and when you were young. What did you do when you felt sad, angry, or scared? If you were like most children, you turned to a trusted adult. These simple yet strong emotions signaled to you that you may need help. Children turn to adults when they experience these emotions.

If you think about it, children come to us because they hope we have answers for them, a solution. They hope that we will *do something* to help them resolve the problems that caused a particular emotion in the first place. Children have a negative emotion because they just had a negative experience, and they come to us because something has *to be done about it*. They may not always know *why* they feel a certain way or *what* has to be done, but they trust we will help them, because their past experience showed them that we can. And we are certainly there to help. And we do try.

Now let's think about what we do when a child is upset.

What is the first place our mind immediately goes to?

We think: the child needs help.

Do we tell them that their negative emotions have caused their negative experience? And do we also tell them that their emotions came from their thoughts?

Of course not.

If, as a child, you have ever been the subject of such treatment, then you know how deeply invalidating and rejecting that feels. And I bet you wished that an adult at least cared enough to ask "What's wrong?" And not in a "What's wrong *with you*" kind of way. Right?

That is exactly what we do when children come to us angry, sad, or scared. We ask them what's wrong. And then we proceed to look for a solution. Sometimes it is about helping them get a turn in a game, finding what's missing, or fixing what's broken, and sometimes it is reassuring them of their safety and offering them comfort.

But something happens when we grow up...

Somehow as adults, when we experience negative emotions, often the first place our mind goes to is — blame. We turn to blaming and shaming ourselves for feeling what we feel. If we do ask questions about our predicament, it is usually something like "What's wrong with me?" as opposed to simply "What's wrong?"

Then we proceed to ignore our emotion, tell ourselves to think happy thoughts, or distract ourselves from it. Some of us will go an extra mile and acknowledge what we are feeling, but then engage in deep analysis of our thoughts to see which ones have prompted our negative emotions. Those of us who are not a fan of what I call "thought-work" may do breath-work or engage in some other form of "mindfulness and presence" to let the emotion "move in and out," as the recommendation goes. Yet we do not offer ourselves this one simple question: "What's wrong?"

What would happen if we did? How would we be able to help ourselves if we approached our own sincere and naturally occurring emotions the way we approach the child's? The key difference is that whereas we see the child's emotions as *natural responses to the world around them*, we look at ours as having no external basis. Same applies when we engage in problem-solving. Whereas when it comes to children, we try to identify what is not working for them and what prompted their feelings, we do not do the same when trying to understand where *our own* emotions come from.

The most important thing to understand is that emotions are valid and purposeful *regardless of our age.* We experience negative emotions because something is *in need of a solution.* Something is not working for us. And so, if we allow ourselves the same inquiry process that we use with children, we may find answers sooner. We may find real solutions as opposed to a temporary relief that may be achieved from dismissing our emotions. With this, let's now turn to the opening questions of this chapter:

W*hat do you do* to process emotions? And if it isn't our thoughts that we have to change in order to feel better, then what is?

The answer becomes simple once we understand where negative emotions come from and what it is that our emotions do. We did talk about that in detail in the previous chapter. So as a quick recap:

Emotions send signals.

They speak.

Emotions speak, and have always spoken to us. As we have previously discussed, emotions are not caused by thoughts, although we can certainly have thoughts about our experience. But even when we have no words, we still have emotions that speak to us about our experience. And that experience can be either a positive or a negative one. When our experience is negative, we have negative emotions. This is the perfect time to ask "What's wrong?" and follow the 3-Step Process I will teach you here.

The bottom line is, we should stop asking: "What's wrong with me?"

Instead, we should be asking "What's wrong?" and be thinking about this question more often than we currently do.

GETTING COMFORTABLE WITH OURSELVES

Before we explore what to do with our emotions and the 3-Step Process to feeling better, let's take a moment to talk about how to get more comfortable with our inner world. Now, why would that be important? Being comfortable with ourselves allows us to really explore what we feel and ask some questions about our emotions, but also find the right answer to what needs to be done about what we feel. That is where the resolution, the answer to the emotions will come from — from within ourselves.

It's rather impossible to be comfortable in our own skin if our emotional experience makes us want to crawl out of it. If you ever wondered why we lack confidence, it is because of the internal discomfort we feel with ourselves. And you know what drives that internal discomfort? Most of the time, it is due to unresolved emotions and difficulty understanding them, which leads to unmet needs. The good news is that once you understand where emotions come from, you will feel so much more comfortable having them and working with them. And no, I will not be telling you to just "accept your emotions" because they are "just a human experience." They are a normal human experience, yes, but there is more to do with it than just be "sitting with it."

Getting comfortable with ourselves starts with *getting to know our inner world* (the world of our feelings, needs, and our thoughts about them). This is where we find ease and confidence. It sounds simple and it is. "Getting to know your inner world" is not just a bunch of words that sound great but bring nothing useful. It is a straightforward sequence of steps, and there aren't many of them.

Only three.

We will get to them in a moment. Without a doubt, the more we know about ourselves, the more comfortable we become. The more comfortable we are, the more confident we feel. Yet we mistakenly believe that we only get to be OK with ourselves when others finally approve of us. Has that ever worked? No. Likewise wrong is the belief that we have to find people who will stop judging us and who will simply accept us. We think that maybe then we will be OK. When we wait for other people to accept us, we waste a lot of time, and miss out on the opportunity to get to know ourselves. Getting comfortable with who we are is not about others and their opinions.

The issue of acceptance is an internal one.

It is about our own relationship with ourselves.

When we are comfortable with ourselves, others naturally respond to that, to our presence, our aura, and our energy. People get comfortable with us *if and when* we are comfortable with ourselves.

The quality of our relationship with ourselves depends on whether we understand our emotions or whether we are at their whim. It is quite impossible to accept who we are if we reject a significant part of ourselves, which is our emotions. When we are living our lives in search of someone else's positive appraisal, what we don't see is the opportunity cost of what we could be doing instead. And that is — getting to know ourselves through our emotions. They tell us what matters to us when we interact with the world. When we understand and appreciate who we are, others will come to appreciate us too. And by that point, you won't even worry about that anymore. Why? Because when we have a deep connection with ourselves, self-acceptance becomes so natural and wholesome, that we don't feel like anything is missing and — naturally — we stop worrying about other people's opinions.

So why do we feel uncomfortable to begin with?

It's because of our emotions. What makes us most uncomfortable with ourselves is our confusing feelings. When we don't understand them or what to do with them, we end up feeling like we cannot trust ourselves. We don't know what to do with ourselves because our emotions overwhelm and confuse us. We also don't like how we act and react when driven by our emotions, which makes us even more stiff and uncomfortable. And so if we are ever to feel comfortable with our internal experience, we've got to change how we process emotions.

Now, we know that things we've been doing before do not work that well (as we discussed in Chapter 1) and we also know that it isn't all in our head (as we saw in Chapter 2), so now what? How do we change the way we process emotions and what does that look like? All of that depends on a clear understanding where emotions come from to begin with, what they are for specifically, and what purpose they serve overall. So let's clarify this next.

THE REAL PURPOSE OF EMOTIONS

Emotions tend to be *the number one obstacle* for many of us. They may feel like a trap we can't wait to get out of. But this is only so when we don't really know what our emotions are for. Do you know what your emotions are for?

They are the key to unlocking our actions.

What kind of actions?

Actions that support our sense of wellbeing.

If we understand our emotions, we can tell what we need to do and what actions we need to take. Emotions contain *so many answers* as to how to make our lives easier, it is ironic how much we try to avoid them! Emotions are there to tell us:

- what we want more of and what we want less of
- what is good for us and what is not so good for us
- what matters to us and what doesn't
- what works for us and what doesn't
- whom to be with and who to stay away from
- what to seek and what to avoid

When we understand the purpose of our emotions, we do what we need to do in order to feel better and feel more like ourselves. When we slow down, pay attention, and listen to our emotions (as opposed to avoid them), we learn to see *what we need*. And in seeing our needs we also learn to see *ourselves*.

Acquiring these emotional skills is truly a game changer.

It gives you the source of energy for the rest of your life. And when I say energy, I don't mean "vibration." You have probably heard others say that emotions are "just a vibration." What is this supposed to mean, practically speaking? When it comes down to it, everything is "just a vibration" because everything is made of atoms that carry molecular vibration, and so this really says nothing.

I find this notion too esoteric, abstract, and — sometimes — misleading. This happens when certain "emotional vibrations" are seen as better than others. There are several "vibrational charts" out there that rate emotions on a scale of high and low, good and bad, and that is just not helpful. Why? Because it devalues the importance and the purpose of the negative emotions, which is to tell us:

- what we want less of
- what is not good for us
- what does not matter to us
- what is not working

Let me tell you right now that the quickest way to feel even more miserable about your emotions is to start judging them as high or low, good or bad. This attitude towards your own emotions will lead to resisting and avoiding them. It is precisely things like this that result in a sense of internal discomfort we discussed earlier. No wonder why this is not helpful.

From the perspective of the real purpose emotions serve (see the bullet points on both pages), it should be clear that emotions have equal value. They don't compete with each other, and don't have a number on a rating scale.

All emotions serve us well and *each one* has a purpose.

Each one requires equal attention and thoughtful action.

As soon as we stop fighting our emotions, our life experiences will significantly improve. We may have been conditioned by our upbringing and previous struggles to believe that emotions make us weak. That is why we hide them and hide from them. Even though it is untrue (emotions do not make us weak), this false belief does make sense, if you think about it, because here is what happens... When we face something powerful, we may — by comparison — feel like we don't measure up, we don't stand a chance. We feel the urge to run, or hide or — if we are feeling brave — to fight it. Truth is, it isn't the emotions that make us weak, but the fight against them that exhausts us. So why do we fight our emotions? Well, the simple answer is because we don't know what else to do and their strength can make us very uncomfortable.

Think of it like Fire.

When the early humans did not understand fire, let alone how to benefit from it, it was scary and destructive. But when they understood what to do with it, it revealed the power to *nurture* (provide warmth, food), to *protect* (against predators), and to *connect* (by creating opportunities for socializing and for prolonged activities into the dark hours of the day). And in that way, humans discovered so much potential in the fire itself and not only did they stop fearing it, they embraced it as a tool. The ability to own fire and use the power of fire took humanity to the next stage of evolution. Instead of running away and feeling inferior to it, we learned how to use it.

We can think about emotions in a similar way. Just like fire, they can be overwhelming and get out of control.

When they are ignored, they can go wild.

To "tame" them we must understand *how*, in addition to seeing their *benefits*. When emotions are noted and understood, they provide us with powerful benefits. They give us nurture and protection, and create possibilities in our life. I do not mean this in a metaphorical way at all, but in a very practical sense. Emotions, when owned and claimed, are the source of your personal strength. They show where your resources are and what to do when those resources are depleted. They are the source of your energy to live your life the way that you want to. Emotions that you can understand and process properly will fuel and support your actions. Meaning, you can show up in your life feeling *nurtured, protected, and connected*. Emotions are the key to our strength, because they tell us *what we need* and *how to get it.*

And so this is what I mean by "energy" in a very down-to-earth way. Instead of thinking of it as "vibration," which I don't find particularly helpful, think of it as *vitality*, a source of *aliveness*, or *personal strength*. You can tell right away when you *don't* have energy — it's when you are exhausted, depleted, and disengaged. You also know when you *do* have energy — it's when you feel engaged or are fully rested. Likewise, you may feel more or less energy depending on what you are doing. Some things feel effortless and some — take a lot out of you to get through.

We can also feel energy *through our emotions*.

This is because emotions reflect the state of our wellbeing. When we are having fun and feel relaxed and happy, we have more energy than when we feel sad or anxious. Why is that? Because these positive emotions tell us that our needs are met and our wellbeing is high. Other emotions show you what drains your energy. And this isn't because some emotions are good and others are bad, but because they show you which parts of your life *work for you* and which ones don't. Emotions show what fills you up and what brings you down or drains your resources. And so this way, emotions reveal to us our resources, which is what meets our needs and gives us energy.

If this is not how you have come to think about emotions, it would be helpful to slow down to process what I am saying. Some of these things need time to sink in. Emotions arise as part of a sophisticated neurological process, which is as crucial and as vital today as it was thousands of years ago. You'll hear people say that our nervous system or the brain is somehow "behind." That our brain sends us false alerts. I say — that is total nonsense. We may not be living in caves or being chased by tigers, but we do have needs, similar to our predecessors.

For as long as we have needs, we will have emotions.

Why? Because the purpose our emotions serve is to let us know whether we are taking care of ourselves and how well we are doing that. Period. It's that simple. Simple and yet complex at the same time. Emotional regulation is the process by which we figure out what kind of help is needed and in what kind of way we need to be taken care of. Emotions let us know what is happening with our needs and resources. Positive emotions tell us that our needs are met and that we have plenty of resources. Meaning, we've got what we need. Negative emotions, on the other hand, let us know that we have unmet needs and that we may also have compromised resources.

So when we don't feel good, it is our emotions' way of telling us we need to do something to meet our needs. And since each one of us is a unique individual, how our needs get expressed through emotions is uniquely ours too (more on that in the next chapter). Not only that, but how our needs are best met is also very individual. That's why getting to know *what* we feel and *why* is the key to getting to know ourselves. This is also why we spend some time talking about getting comfortable with this process.

When we know ourselves, we understand our needs.

When we understand our needs, we can meet them better.

Even though we are sophisticated individuals, we do not have to make things more complicated than they are. And so, even though our emotions can be quite nuanced, it all comes down to signaling whether we are OK. When we feel good, we know we are taken care of and all is well. When we don't, we know that something specific needs to happen to have our needs met. Simple enough, right?

So how do you claim the power of your emotions?

Notice that I am not saying power *over* your emotions. You are not trying to win over an enemy.

You are getting to know yourself and what supports your own well-being. When you see your emotions as an extension of you, you claim them as yours, and you get them to work for you. Much like you would use your hands. They are yours, you put them to work, you take responsibility for what your hands do and you try to make the best use of them. That is what it means to claim your emotions — seeing them as belonging to you and using them in a way that is intentional and beneficial to you. Or another way of saying this would be — using them in an intelligent way. Understanding what your emotions communicate about what you need is what makes you — *emotionally intelligent.*

An emotionally intelligent way of processing emotions has nothing to do with changing our thoughts. That is not how we get to feel better. It's not about what you think, but about *what you need* and also about *what you do* to meet those needs. So let's sort this out and review the 3-Step Needs-Based Emotional Regulation Process (NBER Process™). I developed this simple method to resolve negative emotions by meeting your needs. For the sake of brevity and ease of reading, I will refer to the NBER Process as 3-Step Needs-Based Process and Needs-Based Process, for short.

3 STEPS TO GETTING WHAT YOU NEED

Many people may be aware of their emotions and many are well-versed in emotional vocabulary. Some people can tolerate emotions pretty well and have learned to patiently wait for them to pass. But is that all you do? What else should you do? The awareness of emotions and the ability to name them couldn't be the real answer, could it? We keep wondering about that because deep down we know that we are not quite satisfied with how we regulate our emotions and may feel that something is missing.

So what is the missing piece?

As complex organisms, we require a lot of energy to function. Our ability to function well depends on our wellbeing, on our vitality. That vitality, which we can also think of as "life energy" (i.e., the energy to "do" life, our sense of aliveness), comes from our energy reserves. So then, naturally, we would tend to avoid people, places, and things that drain and consume our energy, and instead seek resources in our environment that help us maintain and restore our capacity. When our energy is low or is unreasonably spent we don't feel great emotionally. Likewise, when we are full of energy, we feel good and our sense of wellbeing is restored into balance.

A critical mistake we make here is that we attribute the source of that energy *to our emotions*, when in fact, emotions simply reflect how we are doing energy-wise (whether we are at high or low capacity). So it isn't proper and will not work to try and elicit certain emotions in hopes that they will give us energy. That is a misunderstanding of the real sources of energy.

It isn't our emotions that give us energy.

It is the *resources* that fulfill our personal needs that do that.

All of the things we have to have in order to function well are expressed through our needs. Needs is something that we all have as living breathing organisms. And as humans, our needs are rather complex, as you might imagine. When our needs are met, we are able to function well and we also feel good. Since emotional regulation is about meeting our needs, how do we get what we need?

We will talk about needs in more detail in Chapter 5, but it is helpful to mention a couple of things about needs here, so that this concept makes sense as we talk about the 3 Steps of the Needs-Based Process to emotional regulation. So what do I mean by "needs" and what kind of needs are we talking about?

Human beings don't just have physical needs. We also have *psychological needs.*

Did you know that?

We are very familiar with physical needs, such as the need for air, for food and water, for rest, etc. When we talk about psychological needs, it is things like the need for safety, the need for control, the need for connection, for meaning, and so on. Psychological needs are just as universal as physical ones, which means all people have them. However, because we are unique individuals, the way our needs are expressed and met is also unique to us.

Negative emotions can be pretty uncomfortable and pretty disruptive. If I were to ask you, what do you need when it comes to negative emotions, what would you say? If you are like most people, you'd probably say — to feel better, to make them less uncomfortable. This answer makes total sense. If we perceive emotions as the cause of discomfort, we would want them to be less uncomfortable. And while I agree, and that this is what you *want*, it is not what you *need*.

What you *need* depends on what your *needs* are.

Understanding our needs is a combination of knowing ourselves and what dynamics in our environment trigger our emotions. This sounds more complicated than it is, and it is something we will explore in Chapter 5, when we talk about needs more specifically. The important takeaway for now is that negative emotions get resolved by looking at the trigger that caused them and attending to the needs they point to. That is why my method is called Needs-Based Processing of emotions, because it directs attention to your needs.

That is the missing piece.

Understanding our needs and meeting them is how we regulate our emotions. So what we have to change when it comes to how we process emotions, is not our *thoughts*, but what we *do*. Our actions in response to our emotions should be directed at meeting our needs. This is very critical to understand. Emotional regulation and the processing of emotions *does not* mean to simply sit with your emotions and it *does not* mean waiting for them to pass. It means to understand *which of the needs is not met* and see what can be done to meet that need. *That and only that* is emotional regulation, and that is the proper way to process feelings.

If all you did was sit with your emotions, feel them in your body, and then wait for them to go away, you missed the point and the purpose. As we discussed in the previous section, the singular purpose of our emotions is to let us know whether we are OK or whether we need to take care of our needs.

With that being said though, the desire to feel less discomfort when it comes to our negative emotional experiences is completely valid. I share it with you, as do most other people. However, what has to happen in order for us to be more comfortable is we have to understand the real source of that discomfort. It does not come from our emotions, it comes from our *unmet needs*. It also comes from our inability to properly resolve emotions, because if we do not understand that emotions point to needs, we will fail to attend to our needs. Consequently, unmet needs lead to unresolved emotions, which perpetuates emotional discomfort.

As we discussed previously, we struggle with this understanding due to lack of knowledge on the one hand and lack of good skills and tools on the other. Although at this point you should have a better understanding about what emotions are for, you still may feel like you don't have the knowledge of how this dynamic (emotions vs. needs) plays out for you. And that is perfectly OK, because we will address each of these things in the chapters that follow.

At this point in our conversation, what I'd like you to have is a bird's eye view of what I am recommending in my 3-Step Needs-Based Process, and after that we will focus on each of the three steps in more detail. It is important not to skip these points because they will frame your perspective around how I recommend regulating and resolving emotions.

It's time you have better tools and better processes.

Although emotional awareness is very important, it is not enough. So let me introduce you to the 3-Step Needs-Based Process that I use personally and highly recommend to others.

In addition to understanding what emotion you are feeling, you also have to be asking yourself two more questions. One of them is — what are your needs? And the other — what could be done to meet your needs? These two questions are the two steps that fill in the missing parts to the emotional regulation process. So what we truly need is to meet our needs. Meeting our needs is how our wellbeing is restored back to a comfortable level. And we get there in three steps, in the following order:

Step 1 ⇒ Emotion Awareness (What are you feeling?)

Step 2 ⇒ Need Awareness (What do you need?)

Step 3 ⇒ Resource Awareness (What should you do about it?)

It's a simple and yet effective process. Now that you know *what* to do, let me show you *how*. I devoted separate chapters to each of these steps, so that we can discuss in detail how each of these pieces work. In the next chapter, we will discuss a couple of simple things you need to know about emotions in order to help yourself when uncomfortable feelings arise.

As I shared with you in the first chapter of this book, one of the reasons why we struggle with emotions is that they have been made too complicated. Well, in staying true with my mission to keep things simple, in Chapter 4 we will only focus on the most necessary things you need to know about emotions. Since this may be the first time you are invited to explore your needs, Chapter 5 will elaborate on this step to help you better navigate needs in general and to understand yours more specifically. And finally, in Chapter 6, we will discuss resources available to you to meet your needs.

One more point I want to make before we move ahead is this: Even though a need is what prompts the signal in the form of emotion and that need occurs first in the sequence of events, it is *the emotion* — and not the need — that we first become aware of.

In other words, the reason why emotional awareness is the first step in the 3-Step Needs-Based Process and awareness of needs is the second step (and not the other way around) is because this is the order in which things appear in our field of awareness. At the same time, it is important to know the true sequence of events, so that we never lose sight of the cause of our emotions, which is — the needs. So even though emotions are what we first become aware of, it is the unmet need that occurs first. Think of it like this: Someone's got to be at the door before they ring the bell, even though we don't know of their presence until the bell rings. It is the sound of the door bell that alerts us to someone's presence. This analogy applies to emotions as well.

Even though things occur like this:

Needs ⇒ Emotions ⇒ Resources

We experience them like this:

Emotions ⇒ Needs ⇒ Resources

And so because we first experience the signal — the emotion — that is where our attention goes first and, therefore, this is naturally the first step in the Needs-Based Process of seeking a resolution to an uncomfortable situation and emotions. At the same time, remembering what comes *before* the emotion and what triggers it, will help you remember *the true purpose* of emotions and keep you on track with that purpose in order to — meet your needs.

If we lose sight of the fact that emotions have a legitimate reason behind them (i.e., our valid and real needs), it is easy to get off-track, thinking things like "What's wrong *with me*?" and "What am I *thinking* that is causing my feelings?" Both of these are not helpful questions, as we have seen earlier.

Since, most likely, this is not the first book you've read about emotions, you may be well-versed in the first step of identifying what you are feeling. And that is wonderful — you are already ahead of the game. Even though you might be tempted to skip the next chapter, here is what I recommend: it is helpful to read all the chapters to better understand how to view emotions in the context of the Needs-Based Process specifically. I promise you — it is very simple. Perhaps even much more simple than what you've heard before and may alleviate some of the extra thinking you may be doing around your feelings. My goal is to strip away the unnecessary complexity so that you feel confident and in control of this simple Needs-Based Process, which only has three steps:

Step 1 ⇒ Become Aware of Your Emotions

Step 2 ⇒ Become Aware of Your Needs

Step 3 ⇒ Become Aware of Your Resources

So as you see, what must change is not the emotions or thoughts, but our actions. And our actions depend on our understanding of our personal needs. Consequently, the steps that we have to take when dealing with discomfort must include understanding and addressing our needs. And that comes from seeing our capacity and resources to meet them.

So let's explore Step One in the next chapter.

Chapter 4

Step One: Emotion Awareness

First, we dismantled the myth that thoughts cause our feelings. Then, we discussed how emotions arise as a signal to a need, rather than as a reaction to a thought. This happens naturally and automatically as a response to something going on in our environment. And so in order to feel better, we have to meet our needs.

Before we are able to figure out what emotions signal to us and what needs in particular do they point at, we first have to be able to detect that signal. That is the First Step in the 3-Step Needs-Based Process of dealing with emotions. We first must be aware of them. So in this chapter we will talk about what these signals feel like, as well as, when and why they may show up.

How do we become aware of our emotions?

We get a sensation of either comfort or discomfort arising within our body. Regardless of what specifically it feels like, we can tell whether it is a good feeling or not. At a very basic level, this is the first phase of emotional awareness. Sometimes, that is all that's needed in order to move on to Step Two, which we will discuss in the next chapter. However, at other times, we can also take it a bit further and become aware of the specific quality and intensity of the emotion to better understand what we feel and what might have caused it. We do this by asking, *what* exactly do we feel, *how* strongly, and *why*?

As humans we are complex beings and, because of that, we experience many feelings. Some of us have words for them and can differentiate between emotions clearly, and some of us may struggle with nuances. Whether we can label them with precision or not, does not change the fact that all of us do experience a wide range of emotions. That is universal amongst humans, whether or not we are clear about what we are experiencing. That means that everyone feels worry, concern, irritation, and so on, even if some of us cannot name that particular feeling.

Naming an experience or labeling an emotion with precision is not necessary in order to have that experience. Naming emotions is also not required in order to know what to do about them. There is plenty of confusing information out there about emotions and, for that reason, I promised to keep things simple. All we need in order to begin, is being able to tell whether the sensation feels positive or negative. So even if you cannot figure out precisely what you are feeling, as long as you can tell whether it is a *positive* or *negative* sensation — which I have no doubt you can — then you will be able to apply the Needs-Based Process I describe in this book.

So let's dive in.

TYPES OF EMOTIONS

Depending on the source, we may be told that there are anywhere from 50 to 150 emotions (and *even more* according to some!). I don't know about you, but I am sure I'd find myself anxious and in despair simply thinking about matching the right label with my emotional experience. This would become especially stressful if I were told that getting the name of the feeling exactly right is a prerequisite to solving my problem. And some experts do tell you that. I disagree.

It's too much pressure.

No need for surgical precision.

Just the idea of going through all the labels would be intimidating. Can you imagine how long the list of 150 emotions is! Instead of instilling a sense of confidence, long lists of feeling words can make us feel unsure of ourselves, wondering whether we are "doing it right," and whether something is badly wrong with us. That's the last thing I want you to do. I don't want you doubting yourself. We want less overwhelm, not more.

And we don't need long lists.

All we need is the basics.

So let's start by differentiating positive emotions from the negative ones.

Positive vs. Negative Emotions

You can do a lot with just this. Even if all you are able to do is differentiate a negative emotion from a positive one, that alone can help you feel better and help you meet your needs, as long as you also ask what your needs are (more on the needs in the next chapter). That sounds pretty doable, right? That's the whole point. This method is designed to be accessible to everyone. Even those who have no knowledge of labels, but can tell whether what they feel feels good or bad, can benefit from the Needs-Based Process. So simple, a child could do it. (Not exaggerating.)

Now, don't get me wrong. Identifying your emotions *is helpful*. However, it is also *not necessary*, and getting stuck on its precise name (worry vs. anxiety, for example) will keep you from resolving that uncomfortable experience. Not to mention, it is energy consuming. Most of our effort should go towards sorting out *what to do* with the emotion as opposed to what specific emotion it is or its precise name. In the simple model that I propose here it is not necessary to differentiate between "stressed" and "overwhelmed," or between "uncomfortable" and "concerned."

Even though we are complex human beings and have nuanced feelings in response to what is happening around us, all of our feelings fall into two main categories — positive and negative. All of our emotions, no matter how long the list, can be divided into either a positive sensation or a negative one, a positive experience or a negative one.

The intensity of any emotion can vary from mild and barely noticeable sensation to very intense. The milder the sensation the more neutral it may feel, and we are less likely to pay attention to it. The more it grows in its intensity, the more urgent it becomes that we attend to it. That is actually the primary reason why emotions grow in intensity, because it is a signal that requires our attention. This variability in how emotions are perceived is what gives them their distinct sensations and their various names.

We will spend less time talking about the positive category of emotions because my guess is you don't need my help there. Most people don't struggle with positive emotions. Unless, of course, they feel guilty about them (more on that in the next section). Generally, positive emotions tell us "all is well." If anything, it would be really helpful for you to notice what happens during those times that make you feel that all is well, so that you can recreate those conditions for yourself again, because they point to what helps you thrive. There are many feelings that fall into this category, but regardless of their specific names and subtle differences, we can simply consider all of them as expressions of wellbeing and "happiness."

Many people take issue with this label, and so I only hold it loosely for the purpose of differentiating positive emotional states (regardless of their nuances) from the negative ones. If you prefer, you can call positive states as simply "pleasant" and falling within the area of *comfort* and vitality. It is when things feel comfortable, at peace, and in balance. Since "happiness" is the word most people are familiar with and since we are not focused on the nuances of positive emotions, this label also works for our purpose here. We are looking for answers as to how to resolve feelings that are *unpleasant* and cause a lot of *discomfort*, and because of that we will spend most of our time on the negative emotions.

It is important to understand that when we look at emotions from the perspective of positive or negative, we are referring to their emotional charge. These are not value labels, and we are not judging them as "good" or "bad." We are only speaking of the way they feel and the message they are sending. That is all. We do not place value on emotions as more or less preferred, because all of them have an equal value in communicating to us about our needs. *All* information surrounding our needs is important and valuable. When things are good and comfortable, our emotions tell us that. That's great to know! Positive emotions tell us what we should seek more of, because that is when our needs are met. Likewise, negative emotions also communicate with us about our needs, except in this case they tell us when things are not good and when we need to take care of something. That, too, is important to know.

Both signals are critical for our wellbeing.

Just as we want to feel a sense of comfort and enjoy our lives, we also want to know when something is wrong. Without that signal we would not know that something needs to be attended to and corrected. Just like we want the fire to give a burning sensation, so as to send us a warning to keep our distance and to be cautious, we also want to be alerted as to which people, places, and things to stay away from. Our emotions will tell us what is good for us and what isn't. What's working and what isn't. That's an important perspective.

You do not have *wrong emotions.*

There are simply things that may be going *wrong around you*, rather than inside you and inside your mind. If you could shift your perspective about emotions and think of them this way, it would hugely benefit you immediately, because it will release a lot of pressure that comes from judging emotions as good or bad, right or wrong.

Think of positive emotions as having a (+) sign, which stands for "yes" and means "needs are met." Likewise, think of negative emotions as having a (—) sign, which stands for "no" and means "needs are not met." If we think about negative and positive emotions in any other way, we may end up running into what is called "secondary emotions." Let's take a look at what that is.

Primary vs. Secondary Emotions

Like I said previously, all emotions are correct and need attending to. We don't have "wrong" emotions. However, when we judge them, we do end up thinking of them in the *wrong way*. If we simply have an emotion, whatever it may be, and not judge it as good or bad, then we simply treat it as *information about our needs*. If needs are met, we appreciate that, and if they are not met — we attend to what needs attending to.

However, if we are judging an emotion as bad, that would make us feel *badly* about having it, which adds an additional layer of complexity. That complexity is called *secondary emotions*. To better grasp what this term means, it helps to understand what *primary emotions* are, because that will give you a good frame of reference. In simple terms, primary emotion is the one that came first and secondary emotion is the one that came second. But there is more to this.

Primary emotions occur as a response to a need, as a *reaction to the environment*. These emotions are spontaneous and precede thoughts. They occur in response to any changes in our environment that may affect the balance of how our needs are being met.

In contrast to that, secondary emotions occur as a *reaction to primary emotions*. Meaning, they occur when we think about our primary emotional reaction and begin to judge it. Depending on our thoughts about the primary emotion and whether we judge it as good or as bad, we will generate additional emotions about it. That is the reason why they are called secondary, because they occur as a secondary response to the emotions that occurred first. Another way of saying it is that secondary emotions are emotional reactions and thoughts *about our emotions*. Whereas the primary ones show up spontaneously in our body as *a reaction to triggers* that have to do with personal needs.

For example, let's say I feel disappointed that it's pouring rain the day I planned to work in the garden. But then I feel bad about myself for feeling disappointed and start telling myself that I should be thinking positively and finding something else to be happy about. So in this scenario, disappointment about the weather is a primary emotion. And disappointment with myself for feeling what I was feeling is a secondary one, because it arose in response to the primary emotion, which I started to judge as a bad one.

Secondary emotions don't reflect our needs, they reflect *our judgments* and, therefore, they are the only emotions that come from thoughts. Secondary emotions often come from overthinking about a problem, ruminating, and judging ourselves, instead of seeing the primary emotion as a valid one and asking how the situation can be helped (i.e., how our needs can be met). When we do not judge our primary emotions, we do not have secondary emotions to deal with. We just focus on the primary emotions to figure out *what* we need and *how* to meet our needs.

Now, secondary emotions can also be experienced as having a positive (+) or a negative (—) charge, depending on whether we approve or disapprove of our primary emotions. The charge expresses whether we like that we feel a particular way or whether we think we shouldn't be feeling that way. More often than not we tend to judge negative emotions and we do that because: a) we do not understand their purpose and b) because we were taught to believe they are no good. But sometimes, it may so happen that we find ourselves judging a positive emotion as a negative experience.

I know this may sound confusing, but hang in there with me.

Remember how earlier I said that most people don't struggle with positive emotions? Typically, we welcome positive emotions and if we were having any thoughts about them — those would produce positive secondary emotions. At the same time, we often tend to judge our negative emotions and shame ourselves for having them. And so it is the negative emotional experiences that are most likely to produce negative secondary emotions. Let's look at some examples of secondary emotions, both as a positive and a negative judgment:

Situation/Scenario	Our Primary Emotion	Judgment/Thought re: Primary Emotion	Our Secondary Emotion
We see our child spill chocolate milk all over his shirt ⇒	Frustration (−)	"I shouldn't be frustrated. He is just a child." ⇒	Disappoint ment (−)
A coworker asks to cover her shift for the N-th time in a row because she is "running late" in hopes we say yes again (because we always have) ⇒	Irritation (−)	"I am so glad I am feeling irritated as opposed to guilty. I am not obligated to do things for others all the time. I should do something about this" ⇒	Proud (+)
Experiencing the beauty of nature during a getaway trip into the mountains. ⇒	Enjoyment (+)	"Wow, I am realizing how much I am enjoying this experience!" ⇒	Happy (+)
Browsing family pictures from the weekend trip (while at work) ⇒	Happiness (+)	"I shouldn't be enjoying this right now" ⇒	Guilt (−)

As with primary emotions, if you like how your secondary emotion feels (proud, happy, etc.), you don't need to concern yourself about changing your perspective. However, if your secondary emotion is negative, this is the time to adjust your perspective about your primary emotions, and also to remind yourself why we have them.

Secondary emotion does not speak to *the need*, but rather it speaks to *your thinking* around emotions you are already having. And so if you are not liking how you are feeling about emotions you are already having, it is because you are *judging them*. So in this case, you need to revisit the previous section to understand that the +/— charge does not mean a good or a bad emotion. It means either the need is met (+) or not met (—), and so we should not be judging and blaming the messenger, which is all that our primary emotions are.

Instead of judging our emotions and, in doing so, generating secondary emotions, it is best we spend our energy figuring out what is not working and how to correct it. So, if we look at the examples on the table above, we would not be judging ourselves for feeling frustrated or irritated. Instead, we would be asking, "What about this situation needs to change?"

- Let's remember that primary emotions are always accurate. They always show us what we need and how to take care of ourselves.

Whatever our opinion may be about them, they carry valuable messages. If our opinion is negative, it does not change the importance of that initial signal. However, our negative judgment about the primary emotion may change what we do about it. Here is what I mean. If we judge and disapprove of our feelings, we may not put effort in resolving what caused them and will miss the opportunity to meet our needs.

Secondary emotions do not add value.

When secondary emotions are negative, they invalidate the original emotional experience, since they try to cancel our initial reaction by disapproving of it. This invalidating effect of the secondary emotional reaction is what leads us astray and far from meeting our needs, because their effect is to dismiss, cover up, hide, ignore, and fight the primary emotion. When that happens, we are not able to complete any of the steps in the 3-Step Needs-Based Process, which starts with awareness and acknowledgement of what we initially feel.

Because of their ability to move us away from meeting our needs, it is critical that you pay attention to any sneaky secondary emotions. Any time you catch yourself criticizing yourself for how you feel, it's a red flag for secondary emotions. Negative secondary emotions do not tend to occur if we accept primary emotions for what they are, attend to them, and respond to the needs they point to. When a secondary emotion shows up, it usually covers up and misdirects our attention away from the original need. And since it takes us away from meeting our needs, when this occurs habitually, it leads to bigger problems, such as unhealthy coping mechanisms.

As we continue the conversation on emotional awareness, let's shift our attention back to the primary emotions. Afterall, these are the emotions that help us live more balanced lives, whereas, secondary emotions don't have much to contribute to us (because they arise from self-judgment and not a need). I just wanted you to be aware of them in case you encounter references to secondary emotions in other contexts.

And so, going forward, all general references to emotions in this book will refer to primary emotions. This is where we apply the 3-Step Needs-Based Process of asking: a) what are we feeling, b) what are we needing, and c) how can we get what we need. If you are still wondering what to do with secondary emotions, stay tuned, because later in the book we will talk more about self-judgment and guilt, and how to resolve them.

THE BASIC TRIAD OF DISCOMFORT

Now that you know the types of emotions we face, let's zoom in and specifically look at how we experience negative emotions. They are the ones that cause us most discomfort and the ones we want to be able to identify in order to sort out what is needed. Out of all the negative emotions you could possibly feel, there are *only three* basic emotions that we truly must grasp in order to address most of our needs.

These three basic emotions are at the core of other negative emotions. Meaning, other, more nuanced, negative emotions come from these basic three. That is why I call them "The Basic Triad of Discomfort." The three emotions that make up the Triad of Discomfort are *Anger*, *Sadness*, and *Fear*.

Each one represents a continuum of feelings that vary in intensity, from mild to moderate to intense. Most other negative emotions will land somewhere along a continuum in either one of these three areas, and they are simply the more nuanced expressions of these Three Basic Emotions. For example, annoyance or frustration are forms of anger that are different in intensity than rage, which is also a manifestation of anger, at the other end of the continuum.

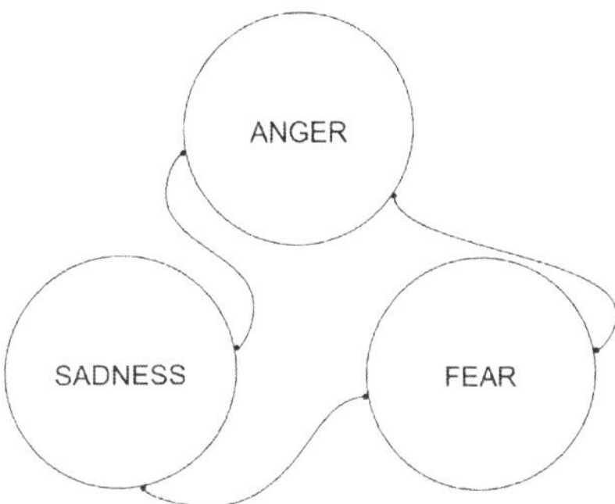

In Appendix A, you will find a table that lists some examples of different ways each of the basic emotions in the Triad of Discomfort can be felt. And although there is quite a bit of variety across feelings within each of the Three Basic Emotions, you will notice that they all share one common quality. In other words, the quality of the primary basic emotion — whether that is Anger, Sadness, or Fear — is evident in all of the feelings listed in that category.

The only difference is the intensity with which these basic emotions are felt on that continuum.

From the perspective of the approach I teach you here, all of these more nuanced feelings can be understood and resolved by applying the same principles used with the three basic negative emotions. Because of that, you don't need to worry about getting your emotions just right or accurately identifying what you are feeling. The only reason I offer to you this expanded list is because you may find it helpful when exploring the nuances of what you are feeling. With that being said, let's briefly walk through each of these three emotions, so that we are on the same page as to what they represent.

Anger

When it comes to *Anger*, this emotion usually rises in response to unfairness. It speaks to a sense of injustice and says "this isn't right," "this isn't fair," or "things shouldn't be this way." It propels us to protect ourselves and our resources, and serves as a call to action to do what's right or fair and to correct things. Anger can range from annoyance to rage.

Sadness

Sadness is an emotion that speaks to an experience of loss. It is a complex emotion that indicates the way we make meaning in the world and calls attention to people, places, and things that have personal significance and feel important to us. We grieve in small and big ways over what truly matters to us. And the deeper the meaning of something we've lost or are about to lose, the deeper the sadness we feel. Sadness can range from wistfulness to despair.

Fear

When it comes to *Fear*, this emotion is an expression of concern for one's wellbeing and safety, as well as the wellbeing and safety of all that which matters to us. Fear is a response to a potential threat to stability and wellbeing. Because of that, it includes an anticipation and an assessment of the potential for a future loss in whatever aspect of our life. Fear can range from caution to panic.

These three emotions are fundamental and basic, which means that the more nuanced feelings can land under the umbrella of one of these three basic emotions. The ease of use with this simple approach is that even if your feelings are rather confusing and complex and you may have difficulty articulating them, you can still get a general sense of what you are feeling. Meaning, at the very least, you will be able to sense whether what you are feeling has the quality of worry (Fear), hurt (Sadness), or whether it has more heat and energy behind it — like Anger.

As long as you can see where in the three general areas your particular emotional experience lands, you will have a sense of how to respond to the emotion and start asking specific questions about yourself and your needs. From there, you can explore the action you have to take in order to meet your needs.

And let me remind you that, even though we simplify things down to just Three Basic Emotions, there is an even simpler approach, which we can call "extreme simplicity." And that is to — simply detect negative feelings, without having to specify what precisely it is or where in the Triad of Discomfort it belongs. Simply noting that you are feeling emotional discomfort *of any kind* is enough to pause and ask:

- What's not right?
- What's not working?
- What am I needing?

This "extreme simplicity" approach helps in cases where emotions are very nuanced and subtle, as well as when you may be feeling more than one kind of emotion. It is also helpful when emotions are too strong and too difficult to deal with, let alone find a proper label for them. You don't ever need to do that. Let's not forget that the main objective of emotional awareness always remains to *detect the need*. It is not as important to identify your feeling "correctly" as it is to *identify your need*.

Identifying a need and then seeking proper resources is where the majority of your effort and energy should go. Knowing what is needed helps us resolve the discomfort, whereas naming an emotion accurately is not enough to help you feel better. It's only the first step.

* * *

Now, you may have noticed that we did not talk about some other emotions that are often mentioned in conversations about basic emotions. These additional emotions are disgust, surprise, and guilt.

There are specific reasons why I am not considering them to be basic emotions and why they are not part of the Triad of Discomfort. So let me say a couple of words about each one of them.

Disgust

This sensation is pretty straightforward and is not at all challenging to detect and decode. We pretty much experience it as a spontaneous reaction to something that we do not align with, something we perceive as harmful for us, something we detest. We are never confused about what it means and we are highly unlikely to judge ourselves for having it. The signals of disgust are strong and clear — to move away and to distance ourselves from what we consider toxic or repulsive. We do not usually engage internally with ourselves to talk ourselves out of it. In terms of where it belongs in relation to other emotions, disgust carries hints of anger and can be placed within that category.

Surprise

I would make a similar point here. Meaning, surprise is another rather straightforward and spontaneous reaction we do not tend to struggle with. It shows up as a reaction to something unexpected and, as such, carries very minor hints of emotions within the fear continuum, in a sense that experiences, which cause surprise, have the quality of startling us or catching us off guard (even when they are fun or pleasant). So if you were wondering where that feeling lands, now you know — within the fear category. It is the emotion of fear in its most mild form — that keeps us vigilant and attentive. Too many surprises, however, and that emotion will grow in intensity, leading us to feeling uncomfortable and perhaps even anxious.

Guilt

This sensation is not a primary emotion at all and for that reason it simply does not belong within basic emotions. It is a form of self-judgment and speaks to concerns about other people's thoughts, judgments, and expectations of us. Still, because guilt does often make us miserable and is something we may feel trapped in, I do address it separately in future chapters. I say "trapped" intentionally here. I say this because guilt does not arise from our own needs and, because of that, there is no resource we can utilize to resolve it effectively. Guilt is driven by other people's needs and our misguided sense of responsibility towards them, but more on that in Chapters 8 and 10.

BECOMING AWARE OF EMOTIONS

Being aware of discomfort is Step One in the Needs-Based Process I am teaching you in this book. We rely on this awareness, so that we can get in touch with our personal needs. Since we want to keep things simple, the only question we will be asking when it comes to negative emotional experiences, is which of the three basic emotions it is. That's it. We will only seek to understand whether it is one out of the three that comprise the Triad of Discomfort, as opposed to searching through a list of countless labels for feelings.

We want to get to resolving emotions and meeting our needs faster, and so it is OK to keep things simple. To understand what we feel, it helps to ask specific questions. You can start by asking:

How am I feeling?

What is coming up for me?

Is something off/not right?

How am I feeling about ______?

It is also OK to ask:

What people, places, or things caused me to feel this way?

This may be an unusual invitation, especially if you were told that emotions do not come from whatever is happening around you. Or, if you were told that places and things are neutral (which, by the way, is only true *sometimes*) and cannot cause an emotion. Or, if you were told that people cannot "hurt your feelings" or trigger an emotional reaction. They most certainly can! If another person's action gets in the way of you meeting your needs, you will most certainly have a reaction, to be sure. And so, it is OK to ask: "What people, places, or things caused me to feel this way?"

Emotions *do* arise in response to our environment, as well as in response to the people and things in it. It is usually some change around us that prompts or triggers either a negative or a positive emotional reaction in order to make us aware of our needs (as we have discussed earlier). And so asking about People, Places, and Things can help us understand what prompted the feeling, and can also help us understand what it is we feel.

Your answer will sound something like:

I feel X because of Y.

Or:

Because Y happened, I feel X.

Sometimes the feeling may be unclear until we examine the trigger. And that is the reason why it is often helpful to ask *what caused* the feeling. For example, I may be feeling awful, which is a general sensation of discomfort, but not sure why. As I start asking questions about potential triggers and see what may be causing me to feel this way, let's say, I realize that it is me sitting in a traffic jam that is making me worried about getting to my destination on time.

No, it is not my thought about being late that is causing the worry (see our discussion about thoughts in Chapter 2), but the potential "threat" to my wellbeing in my environment that is doing that. What is that threat in this particular situation? It is the traffic and the amount of time lost in it. Meaning, I am concerned and worried about losing time and being late. Losing time is a legitimate concern, particularly when we are short on time (and especially in our fast-paced world).

Now, a threat does not need to be severe (such as a threat to life) in order to upset our internal balance. Anything that is compromising or has the potential to compromise our wellbeing, be it in minor or major ways, is a threat to our wellbeing. The intensity of our emotions indicates the magnitude of this impact that specific situations have on us.

We may be jumping slightly ahead here, but I do want to point out that in this example we see several things come together in terms of the 3-Step Needs-Based Process to dealing with emotions. In this example, you see how a *trigger* (which is — sitting in traffic) helped identify the *emotion* of worry (which falls within the Fear category). And that emotion helped us identify the *need* — of getting to the destination on time. What I want you to note is that the need "to get to my destination on time" is what caused the emotion, not some thoughts I may have about the traffic. My wellbeing was threatened because of the conditions in the environment that were compromising my ability to meet that need.

To resolve this situation fully, the remaining step here would be to seek appropriate ways to meet the need, which is something we address when we talk about resources in Chapter 6. This is another place where asking the question "What people, places, or things caused me to feel this way?" can point to the right solution, the right resource. You will see this play out as we move through Step Two and Step Three.

To get in touch with what type of emotion we are feeling, more specifically, we can ask even more questions. Answers to these additional questions can pinpoint which of the three basic emotions — Anger, Sadness, or Fear — we are experiencing.

We can "scan" our mind for cues and we can also scan our body for additional signals. Start with the following questions for both, mind and body, and see which one resonates with you the most. And, of course, if you already have clarity as to which of the three emotions in the Triad of Discomfort you are feeling, you do not need to ask these additional questions.

To access cues from your mind, do a "Mind Scan" by asking the following questions, or some version of them:

1. *Does something seem unjust or unfair?*
2. *Did I/will I miss or lose something? Is something gone?*
3. *Am I concerned something bad will happen?*

As you reflect and tune into the answer, notice what comes up. If you answered "yes" to the first question, your feeling belongs to the emotional category of Anger. If you answered "yes" to the second set of questions, the feeling you are feeling is within the Sadness category. And the final question points to feelings within the Fear category.

For cues from the body, do a "Body Scan" by asking these questions and tuning into your internal sensations for answers:

1. *Does my body energy feel warm or hot?*
2. *Does the energy in my body feel low or heavy?*
3. *Does my body energy feel antsy? Perhaps, chilled or cold?*

If you answered "yes" to the first question, your sensations are consistent with emotions on the Anger continuum. If you answered "yes" to the second question, the sensations you are feeling are consistent with the emotion of Sadness and other related feelings. And if you answered "yes" to the final set of questions, those sensations point to the emotions within the Fear continuum.

Typically, your sensations from the body will align with the answers from the mind. If not, that may mean you have several conflicting emotions, which is totally normal too. It simply speaks to the complexity of your situation, and each of the emotions will have to be attended to separately.

Here is a quick easy-access reference to the *Mind/Body Scan* questions we just discussed:

Mind Scan	If "*YES*"	Body Scan
– Does something seem unjust or unfair?	Anger	Does my body energy feel warm/hot?
– Did/will I lose something? Is something gone?	Sadness	– Does my body energy feel low or heavy?
– Am I concerned something bad will happen?	Fear	– Does my body energy feel antsy, chilled, or cold?

If we are not used to checking in with ourselves this way, it may take some practice asking these questions until we get to know ourselves. That way we will learn how different emotions show up and feel in our body, as well as the kinds of thoughts that tend to float in our minds that help point to specific triggers.

You could also practice this approach retroactively, by recalling specific situations from the recent past, where you know exactly how you felt. Can you think of a situation that happened some time earlier today or this week that made you feel either angry, or sad, or worried? Revisit those situations in your mind and see how the Mind/Body Scan questions align with what you experienced.

It may be that our sensations are so nuanced and subtle (such as, irritation, for example) that it is difficult to tell what we are feeling and whether anything needs to be done about it. That is OK.

The more practice we have, the easier it will be to detect our emotions early on and respond to them proactively, in a timely way. However, in the early stages of learning to sense and understand our emotions, we may be only picking up on emotions that have higher intensity (such as, frustration). And that is OK. You are not missing out on anything. Our internal system of navigation — our emotions — is designed to "up the ante" so to speak if the more subtle signals are missed. So if you miss the feeling of mild irritation and ignore the need behind it, it will grow in intensity to something *you will* notice — such as feeling quite bothered or frustrated.

Before we move on and talk about needs, let me make a note here that *missing the signal* is not the same as noticing it and yet *deciding to dismiss it* as not important. This tends to happen when we judge emotions as worthy of our attention or not, as good or bad, or as a nuisance as opposed to as something important.

Deciding to dismiss an emotion also points to an attitude problem in regards to how emotions are perceived generally and what beliefs we have about them, which is something we talked about in the very first chapter. And as we discussed, emotions are signals we do not want to miss, let alone *dis*-miss, because they speak to us about what we need. And, if we want to feel better on a regular basis, we simply must get better at taking care of ourselves and our needs.

Emotions remind us to look after ourselves.

And with that, let's talk about what our needs are.

Chapter 5

Step Two: Need Awareness

We live in a culture that advocates well on behalf of others, but not on our behalf. We are strongly encouraged to donate, contribute, give, attend, and serve — all of which are wonderful things — but without taking a minute to reflect on whether we have our own needs met.

And that's where the problem is. Although we are told to care for others, we are not usually taught how to find energy for that or how much of that is actually our personal obligation. We are also not taught to understand that our primary responsibility is — ourselves.

It is *our* responsibility to meet *our* needs.

Our emotions remind us of that on a daily basis.

As they say, where there is smoke, there is fire. Since we are talking about emotions, we would say — where there is a Feeling, there is a Need. The most uncaring thing we can do to ourselves is to dismiss our feelings, and do so repeatedly. This may sound harsh, but it's true, because in doing so we end up dismissing our needs.

Consequently, what that does, is we are unable to meet them. When we blow on the smoke in hopes of it going away, we might make it move and it may appear less intense. However, it does not take care of the fire that feeds it. To clear the smoke, we need to put out the fire. As it applies to emotions, we would say — to take care of the feeling, we have to take care of the need that generated it. And to take care of our needs, we have to understand what they are.

A fundamental shift that is required in our perspective is realizing this:

- It isn't our emotions that make us unhappy, but our unmet needs.

One of the ways we neglect our needs is by dismissing our emotions. Another way we do that is when we misattribute the cause of our emotions. So many of us were taught that emotions come from thoughts (a myth we debunked earlier). If we believe something like that, we end up working hard on changing our thoughts in order to feel better, and in doing so we miss the opportunity to meet our needs, which is the actual source of our emotions.

Instead of working hard on changing emotions or shifting our thoughts, what we have to do is — change our actions in a way that helps us meet our needs. The steps that we have to take when dealing with emotional discomfort must include understanding and addressing our needs. And how focused and intentional our actions are will depend on our understanding of what we need.

We have to move from Step One — Emotion Awareness (i.e., a realization that something is causing us discomfort), to Step Two — Need Awareness (i.e., finding what's out of balance). In order to understand what we need and to be aware that *there is* a need, we must first pay attention to our emotions. Which is why, if you haven't explored Step One that we discussed in the previous chapter, please make sure you do.

Since emotion is a signal that tells us something is requesting our attention, then we have to ask *what's needed*. Emotions arise as a reaction to our environment (contrary to what we have been taught traditionally). That is what they are for — to alert us to something going on around us that may or may not be serving us and that — when it comes to signals from negative emotions in particular — is compromising our wellbeing. *Our wellbeing depends on the balance of our needs.* When our needs are out of balance or when we are out of sync with our needs, we don't feel our best or in harmony with ourselves. And that ends up being expressed in one of three basic emotions in the Triad of Discomfort.

Unpleasant emotions resolve
when we get what we need.

They don't resolve if we just wait for them to go away, nor do they go away if we simply *pretend* they are not there. Quite the opposite. When needs are not met and go unmet repeatedly, it leads to more unpleasant emotions (often of higher intensity). If we don't see needs behind our feelings, we will resort to distracting ourselves from them. And when we hide from what we feel, we miss out on resources that can meet our needs and make us feel in-harmony with ourselves, balanced, and content.

We will talk about resources and how to meet our needs in Step Three, which is discussed in the next chapter. First let's make sure you have a good understanding of the range of human needs, so you can be aware of them and begin to notice them in yourself.

TYPES OF HUMAN NEEDS

All living things have needs. These needs have to be met in order for the organism to survive. Depending on the complexity of that organism, the needs vary from very basic to nuanced and sophisticated. Since this isn't a lesson in biology, I am going to oversimplify and say that plants need sunshine, animals need air, fish need water, and so on. You get the idea. Everything that is alive, that grows and changes — has needs of its own.

When these needs are not met, the wellbeing of that animal or plant is threatened. Because of that, each organism has built-in mechanisms and sensors to detect and respond to the needs in order to help that organism thrive and prolong its survival. Even a flower will twist and turn to get the most out of the sunshine available. Certain species of birds and fish migrate as seasons change to places where the living conditions are most comfortable and appropriate for them. Isn't nature amazing!

Now, we are not like the other organisms and our needs do definitely differ. Given the complexity of human beings, one can expect that the needs we have will be multifaceted and complex too. Likewise, our built-in mechanism of detecting needs and responding to them is also more advanced compared to other creatures.

We are very familiar with our physical needs such as the need for air, for food and water, for rest, warmth, etc. Physical needs are the needs of the body. And we are generally pretty good at meeting these needs.

Some of us are less intentional and thoughtful about how we go about it than others, but even so, most of us do not go on completely neglecting our physical needs. This is because all of us (unless something is wrong with our functioning) are adept at registering the signals that our body sends us and then respond to those signals accordingly. When we are hungry, we eat. When we are tired, we rest. When we are cold, we do something to increase the sensation of warmth.

Speaking of complexity...

Human beings don't just have physical needs.

We also have *psychological needs.*

Physical needs are relatively straightforward and simple to understand. But what do you think of when I say "psychological needs"? What are they? Simply put, psychological needs are the needs of the mind. And when I say "mind" I mean the complex parts of our being that make us human and that go beyond the body and the brain. It is everything that has to do with our Self, and so we will refer to psychological needs interchangeably as the needs of the Self. The mind, or the Self, represent everything that makes us uniquely human and, thus, different from all other living organisms. It is our consciousness, our psyche, our soul... — all the many ways in which we think about the mental and spiritual parts of ourselves.

As you can imagine, these needs can and do encompass a lot of things. It is everything that makes us unique beings that we are.

The point is not to debate the accuracy of these terms or to agree on how to differentiate "mind" from "consciousness" or "psyche" from "spirit" and so on. Opinions and schools of thought vary when it comes to definitions, and that is not our focus here. The only matter of importance to us in this book and for the purpose of resolving emotional distress is to understand that we have *a wide range of personal needs*, and that they extend far beyond our physical needs.

With that in mind, and for the sake of simplifying this rather complex set of needs, anything that does not directly correspond to the needs of our Physical Bodies falls into the category of our Psychological Self. And going forward we will interchangeably refer to physical needs as "*the needs of the Body*" and refer to psychological needs as "*the needs of the Self.*"

Our psychological needs are not only very different from our physical needs, they also vary in intensity and scope based on who we are as individuals. Here is what I mean. Psychological needs are universal, which means all people have them. Just like all people have the needs of the Body, each person will also have the needs of the Self. However, because we are unique individuals, the way psychological needs are expressed is also unique to us. And because the expression of our psychological needs is unique to us personally, we will have individual differences in how we go about meeting them, just like we all differ in how we meet our physical needs. In other words, although everyone has physical needs, everyone's body is different. Some people feel cold when others don't. Some people need more food than others, and some have allergies, while others don't, and so on. Likewise, although all of us have psychological needs, the way they show up for us individually will be different from the way they show up for others.

Here is what's very important to pay attention to: When it comes to our needs, we are more likely to meet our physical needs than we are to attend to our psychological needs. And that is what makes processing emotions such a challenge for us. Let me explain.

One of the reasons why we are less likely to attend to the needs of the Self is our level of awareness around those needs. We all understand that we need to eat, sleep, move, etc. We register and understand signals from our body that tell us when our body has a need. But not so when it comes to psychological needs. Another reason why we are less likely to attend to them is that we have developed habits and intentions around our physical needs and do not tend to think twice about meeting them. But when it comes to psychological needs, not only we may not be aware of what they are, we may also *miss the signals* that tell us a psychological need is present.

Psychological needs *are not* secondary to our physical needs.

They are *just as* important.

Both sets of our needs work in tandem to ensure our wellbeing. This is so because we are not just our bodies, we also come with higher consciousness than any other creature we know. Habitually we tend to acknowledge the needs of the body and ignore or not be aware of the needs of the Self (i.e., psychological needs). We have to learn to acknowledge their existence and sense their presence.

But how do we sense their presence, you may ask. Whereas specific sensations in our body (such as hunger, thirst, pain, etc.) tell us about the needs of the body, *emotions* are the ones that alert us about psychological needs. Emotions are the sensations that signal whether or not our psychological needs are met. We feel positive emotions when our needs are met and negative emotions — when they are not.

And just like emotions are universal to all human beings, but their expression (when and why they show up) is unique to each one of us, the same is true for our psychological needs. They are universal, but their expression is unique to each one of us. I am repeating this so that we drop the judgment around them. If we judge our needs, we will dismiss them as too frivolous, a sign of privilege, something to avoid or to overcome.

Meeting our needs ensures our wellbeing.

When we ignore our needs, we suffer.

Understanding the complexity and the range of our needs ensures that we attend to all of them, not just the needs of the body, but also the needs of the Self. Before we discuss the kinds of psychological needs we have and what our emotions may be pointing towards, let's make sure you understand that needs are OK to have.

Since we have a tendency to dismiss our emotions or struggle with them, we rarely understand the needs they point to. And because of that, along with emotions getting a bad rap, our psychological needs may also be frowned upon. In fact, as you read this chapter, you may be noticing a judgment arise within you in regards to psychological needs. This would be especially true for those of us who habitually neglect what we need and desire. Some of us don't want to be perceived as "being needy" or being seen as having "unresolved issues." That is understandable given our culture and lack of awareness around how critical psychological needs actually are to our wellbeing.

However, the only time where that expression ("being needy") makes sense is when we expect others to take care of our needs and become a burden to them. We will talk about that more later on. But for now let's just be clear that there is nothing wrong with having our own needs and attending to them, as long as we go about it in the right way. We will talk about what this looks like in just a bit.

Calling anyone out for having psychological needs is as unfair as telling them they should be ashamed for needing to sleep, eat, or use the bathroom. Would we do this to a friend? Would we judge them for having needs? This sounds pretty ridiculous when I am using physical needs as an example. However, we do that all the time when it comes to psychological needs, especially our own.

Would we tell a child to "stop being needy" when they want to play? Would we neglect a pet that is needing something? Do we judge a plant for needing more space, or sun, or water?

Nope, no, and never.

Then why do we do this to ourselves?

We judge our emotions.

We judge our thoughts.

And we neglect the full spectrum of our needs.

If, in addition to having a negative perception about our emotions, we also judge ourselves for having needs, then how likely is it that we will be intentional about meeting them? Highly unlikely. And since negative emotions arise in response to unmet needs, how likely are we to feel miserable eventually? Very likely. To prevent this outcome, we have to understand our needs and meet them intentionally, regularly, and proactively.

You've probably heard before that it is OK to really feel your emotions. Although some of us do need a permission like this, it is not enough. It is time we give ourselves another permission and that is —

the permission to take care of our needs, instead of shying away from them.

In order to understand that both types of needs are OK, we simply have to acknowledge that *we are more than our bodies.* We find meaning in things, we care about what's important to us, we need to laugh, to have connection, a sense of security and fulfillment. These don't come from food, shelter, rest, etc. Our psychological needs cannot be met the same way that we meet our physical needs. Drinking water will make us less thirsty but it will not stop us from pursuing meaning. Having food will curb hunger, but will not give us a sense of fulfillment.

Our belly may be full but our heart — empty.

You get the idea.

Every day we exert energy, no matter what we do. Not only do we exert physical energy, but psychological as well. And this is especially true when we interact with other people, who may come with their own needs and emotions, and can have an impact on how we feel. So we may be exerting even more energy than we are aware of. Interacting with the world around us takes up a lot of our internal resources (both physical and mental), which is OK, so long as we remember to restore them.

Just like being hungry or sleepy does not make us a bad person, it only indicates that we have a need to restore physical energy, same goes for our psychological needs. They are real and require attention. Experiencing the feeling of emotional depletion does not make us bad people, it just signals to us that we have neglected our own psychological needs and have to find ways to meet them. Unlike with physical needs, sometimes we forget to fulfill our psychological needs and to restore back to our own baseline of being nourished and balanced mentally, emotionally, and spiritually.

The resources required to meet the needs of the Self are very different from the ones required to meet the needs of the body. We will talk more about that in the next chapter. The bottom line is that we have both types of needs and we have them because we are *alive* in the most encompassing sense of this word. Consequently, if we want to feel *fully alive*, we have to attend to the whole spectrum of needs of our being. When we don't, we feel uneasy, disconnected, unfulfilled, and even "dead inside" as some would say.

In order to do our needs justice, we also have to understand that they are ongoing and ever-present. Meeting them regularly is what sustains us, what keeps us going on a daily basis. We don't just eat one meal and are done eating altogether. We don't expect one breath to carry us through the day either.

Psychological needs are like that too. They get met and, soon after, they have to be met again. Understanding what our needs are, how they show up, and what works for us in order to meet them, is when we strike a good balance and feel present, grounded, and fully alive.

CORE PSYCHOLOGICAL NEEDS

All of our needs are an expression of who we are as human beings, and meeting our needs allows us to *be well* and to *be ourselves*. Just like all humans have shared physical needs, all of us have common psychological needs, all of which are a reflection of what it means to be a human being. Because every person has the same kinds of needs and these needs are universal (meaning, common amongst all people), I call them "core" as they are at the core of what makes us human. They are at the core of our *being*. Therefore, they are fundamental to our *well-being*.

In other words, they are essential to our sense of vitality, to our survival. If we neglect our psychological needs, all we have is a walking body with no consciousness, no soul, no light. There are many ways to describe what happens to individuals who only attend to their physical needs. You get the point.

To make it easier to see the range and the scope of our psychological needs, I have divided them into eight broad categories. Many different expressions of the same kind of need will fall within each category. And so, although we are all unique and the expression of each of these 8 Core Psychological Needs is unique to us, it will still fall within either one of these categories. Not only are our needs and their expression unique to us, but also is the way we meet them, which we will discuss in the next chapter when we talk about Step Three. What satisfies my needs is different from what satisfies your needs in each of these categories. However, all of us have needs in each of these domains of psychological functioning.

So let's take a look at each one of these 8 Core Psychological Needs, so you can gain a better awareness of them. Although they appear on the page in a certain order, I want you to know that this order is random and that our needs don't have a hierarchy. Each one is just as important to attend to as another. The only needs that have priority over others are the ones that are unmet at any given moment.

Safety & Comfort

One of our Core Psychological Needs is the need for Safety & Comfort. Now, this is not to be confused with safety and comfort that our *body* needs, but the safety and comfort that applies to us *as a whole person*.

This manifests as the need for privacy, stability, predictability, and the sense of comfort in your own skin so to say. It includes a need for private time and having opportunities to be one-on-one with ourselves. It also refers to being able to trust others and ourselves, as well as to feel secure within ourselves and our relationships. This also has to do with the need to have some of our thoughts and experiences private, kept to ourselves, and having boundaries around what we are willing and wanting to share. Without these things we feel exposed and vulnerable.

You can pause and take a minute to reflect, how does this core need show up for you? What do *you* need in order to have the sense of Safety & Comfort with yourself and in your relationships?

Freedom & Autonomy

Next let's look at our need for Freedom & Autonomy, which is an expression of what we call Free Will. This category of needs includes such necessities for our functioning as independence, sovereignty, self-determination, self-sufficiency, and so on. These needs, when met, allow us to express our individuality and pursue personal goals, have preferences, form our own opinions and have our own vision.

We see this need for Freedom & Autonomy manifesting naturally throughout the progression of human development and various life stages. For example, it shows itself in things like when the child says "Me, me, me. I do it!" to insert their independence. As we get older, we do have the same need and, although it will manifest itself slightly differently, it does not go away. It is this need that helps us set good boundaries to protect ourselves from unwelcome influences. It also shows up when we feel "managed" and "micro-managed" by someone. Having autonomy is core to our nature of being individuals, being *separate* from others.

Take a moment to reflect, how does this core need show up for you? What do *you* need in order to have the sense of Freedom & Autonomy?

Agency & Control

The need for Agency & Control expresses our need to feel strong, capable, reliable, trustworthy, and in control, and it is closely related to our need for Freedom & Autonomy. We take pride in our ability to do things without other people's assistance, which helps us feel like we can rely on ourselves and count on ourselves, because this gives us a sense of control. Deep down it is our innate calling to have a sense of self-reliance, as opposed to feeling dependent on others.

When we depend on others, we are not free, which taps into our need for Freedom.

This category of needs speaks to wanting to feel impactful, to have personal power and strength, to carry a sense of personal responsibility, and to respond to the demands of our lives to the best of our ability. To the extent that is meaningful and applicable to us, it can be expressed through things like achievement, leadership, pursuit of goals that express who we are, and support our sense of strength and accomplishment. It is similar to when the children proudly show off what they did ("Look, I did all of this by myself!") and have a sense of pride in their skills and abilities. We want to achieve things, to feel our own ability and capacity to have an impact on our life, and to preserve what matters to us.

Here too, I invite you to reflect about the ways in which this core need shows up for you. What do *you* need in order to have the sense of Agency & Control?

Worth & Acknowledgment

The need for Worth & Acknowledgment has to do with our need to be seen and heard, to know that we matter, that we are valuable individuals, and that we are worthy. This need, like all other ones, can be satisfied in many ways. For example — being attended to, being appreciated for who we are, being heard and understood, being recognized for our accomplishments, having worth in our own and other people's eyes, being valued, etc. — are just some of the ways in which we can feel seen and like we matter.

Depending on who we are or the season in our life, we may meet this need through getting attention from others or gaining a particular status in a group, and at other times we may prefer to meet it through a deeper connection within ourselves and through our own self-acceptance. If you have a spiritual practice that serves and supports you in deeply nourishing ways, it is most likely because it teaches you to appreciate yourself and see yourself as a worthy being who matters.

So take a minute to reflect, how does this core need show up for you? What do *you* need in order to have a sense of Worth & Acknowledgment?

Fun & Enjoyment

The need for Fun & Enjoyment is another basic human need and it is probably the one you will feel most familiar with. It's that spark you we all know, especially when it's missing. Most of us can relate to a feeling that comes from not having enough fun and enjoyment in our lives. And most of us can find many ways to satisfy this need. This core category speaks to our need to have spontaneity, playfulness, and carefree moments of ease and enjoyment in our lives on a regular basis. It is essential that we have moments of delight for no other reason than to fill our hearts with joy.

And of course, just like with other needs, what is fun and enjoyable for each one of us will be unique to us personally. Because of that, what we will need in order to have this need met, will differ from person to person.

How does this core need show up for you? What delights you? What do *you* need in order to have a sense of Fun & Enjoyment in your life?

Stimulation & Growth

The need for Stimulation & Growth speaks to our pursuit of challenges that help us grow and evolve in many different ways that are personally meaningful to us. It speaks to our innate curiosity and desire to learn. In order to evolve and continue to develop throughout our life span, we need to stretch beyond the comfort of what we already know. It is important to strike the right balance so that the newness and the stimulation are not exceeding what we need at any given moment. Otherwise, it will feel like too much to handle and will become overwhelming. And so this aspect of this need is complementary to the need for Safety & Comfort, which helps us strike the right balance between how much growth is manageable for us at any stage of our lives.

In other words, as we venture outside of our comfort zone to meet our need for Stimulation and Growth, we also have to balance that with the need for control and to ensure we are doing that safely. This way, whatever new things we are learning and all the areas in which we are growing, feel manageable and beneficial, as opposed to overly scary and threatening, which will only lead to anxiety. And again, how we do that, will be unique to our personality and individual expression of our needs.

Take a moment to think about how this core need shows up for you. What do *you* need in order to have the sense of Stimulation & Growth?

Connection & Intimacy

The need for Connection & Intimacy speaks to relationships in general, with other people, with ourselves, pets, and even beyond (as in, feeling connected to Nature, God, Higher Power, etc.). We have a need to feel a part of something, whether that is something close to heart and small or whether it is rather grand but still intimately personal. This stems from the desire to not be alone, to have a sense of companionship in this world, something that holds us grounded and tethered in all the good solid ways. Without that, the world may seem too big, too cold, distant, and overwhelming.

We have a natural need for belonging and to form attachments with those who matter to us. We have the need to feel and experience those things with care. Some of these connections are deep and highly intimate, and some less so. And when we speak of intimacy, it represents closeness and the depth of that relationship. It is the degree to which we feel connected to someone or something. Closeness is a big range of experiences that include but are not limited to physical closeness, interpersonal closeness, emotional closeness, intellectual connection, a sense of deep spiritual connection, and so on.

So what about you? How does this core need show up for you? What do *you* need in order to have the sense of Connection & Intimacy?

Meaning & Purpose

The need for Meaning & Purpose is perhaps the one that most uniquely illustrates how special and complex we are as human beings. Because we have inquisitive and creative minds, we want to know the reason, the bigger Why of our lives. We ask questions about the world around us and how it works, but we also ask similar questions about ourselves and our actions. We want to know that what we do matters, that it has meaning and purpose. When it comes to purpose, this need can be expressed in smaller ways, such as making specific actions and tasks purposeful, and making sure that what we do on a daily basis makes sense to us. But it also expands into the realm of more existential questions, such as what is one's purpose in life, which may lead to a life-long inquiry and a profound personal journey.

When this need is met, we can have a sense of impact and contribution in the world, but more importantly a deep sense of satisfaction from a life that feels meaningful. And because all of us are different human beings, what we find meaningful and important varies. Where we find our sense of purpose and fulfillment is also very individual.

As we conclude this list, take some time to reflect — how does this core need show up for you? What do *you* find meaningful in your life? What do *you* need in order to have a sense of Meaning & Purpose?

There you go! These are the 8 Core Psychological Needs. And here is a list of them, all in one place (in no particular order):

- Safety & Comfort
- Control & Agency
- Freedom & Autonomy
- Worth & Acknowledgment
- Fun & Enjoyment
- Stimulation & Growth
- Intimacy & Connection
- Meaning & Purpose

We will continue to reference them throughout the book, and so it may be helpful to take a peek at Appendix B, where you have all the needs at a glance. As I mentioned, these are eight broad categories of psychological needs that encompass their more nuanced expressions, which are unique to who we are as individuals. Hence, the questions I invited you to reflect upon within each core need category.

To take care of ourselves means to take care of our personal needs, which go beyond physical needs and include these psychological needs as well. We all have them, even though the way they are expressed may differ from person to person. And, consequently, how they are met will differ from one individual to another, as we shall discuss in the next chapter.

One important point I want to make here is that there is a difference between psychological needs and what you may hear others refer to as "emotional needs." Though I do not find this concept particularly helpful, I would like to explain it nonetheless, so that when you hear it, you know where to place it. It also helps you orient yourself within the Needs-Based Process and not lose sight of what is important.

The easiest way to think of "emotional needs" is to think of it as the need to be seen and heard, especially during emotionally changed events. Considering the 8 Core Psychological Needs we reviewed, this is a manifestation of our core need for Worth & Acknowledgement.

Since emotions create a strong personal experience, it is asking to be acknowledged and validated (either by ourselves or others) as an important one. And it is typically within the context of emotional experiences that you will usually hear this reference to "emotional needs." Because of this narrow angle, I find the term limited and not fully reflective of the whole range of psychological needs. So when you hear someone talk about "emotional needs," just remember that the needs of the Self go way beyond the need of acknowledgment and validation.

Now that we know what our psychological needs may look like, let's talk about how to become aware of our needs as they come up.

THE "WHAT'S WRONG?" INQUIRY

Unmet needs let themselves be known through uncomfortable or negative emotions. As we register that emotion (Step One: Emotion Awareness), we can move into Step Two, which is Need Awareness, and ask ourselves what need is coming up. In a much simplified way, this looks like asking ourselves: "What's wrong?" Yes, that very same question we discussed several pages ago. We ask this question with curiosity and compassion, not with judgment.

We ask to find out, not to dismiss.

If our tone (yes, we do speak to ourselves with a particular tone) is exasperated or judgmental, we will not learn anything about ourselves and what we may be needing. And that will only mean one thing — we will fail to identify the need behind our emotion. If we don't identify the need, we will fail to meet it. When we ask "what's wrong?" our goal is to find out what is not working, so that we can do something about it. That way we meet our needs and bring back the balance.

We can ask even more questions, depending on the kind of emotion we are feeling. Even just working with the three basic emotions (the Triad of Discomfort) can reveal a lot about what may be going on for us in any given situation.

For example, if we are feeling anger, we can ask — *What's not right or fair? What is it that am I trying to protect, fix, or get back?* If we are feeling fear, we can ask — *What do I think will happen? What am I concerned about?* And if we are feeling sadness, we can ask — *What didn't work out? What has been lost? What was important?*

The answers behind each of these questions could point to something small or big, based on our needs, perspectives, and personal meaning that specific situations and things have for us. For example, when it comes to sadness, we may be feeling disappointed over canceled plans with a friend (a relatively small issue, because we can make new plans) or be completely devastated when someone cheated on us (a big deal, because it means a loss of a whole relationship as we know it).

Notice that when I say "small or big" I am not suggesting that we judge these events as important or not important and, therefore, decide whether to dismiss them. Not at all. They already have importance, and the way we know this is because we have feelings about them. If they were not important, we would not have an emotional response to them. The magnitude of impact, and therefore the magnitude of our emotional response, dictates the kind of resources that will be required to address the need.

In the first example, since our emotion of disappointment over canceled plans may signal to us that we still want to see our friend, we will meet our needs by making new plans. In the second example, however, we may have to reflect on what that relationship meant to us, how it impacts our sense of Self, how we can rebuild trust in ourselves and others, etc. As you can see, addressing the needs prompted by that experience, is a much more involved process. It will take some time and reflection to find the proper resources to deal with a situation of that kind.

In the previous chapter we talked about the traffic jam example. We discussed how a *trigger* (which is sitting in traffic) helped identify the *emotion* of worry. We also identified the *need* behind that emotion, which was getting to the destination on time. That awareness of the need came from asking questions like "Why am I feeling worried? What is making me worried? What's not working for me here? What matters to me?"

By the way, you may be noticing that "being on time" was not mentioned in the 8 Core Psychological Needs. That is because those core needs are broad categories that represent more specific expressions of needs such as, for example, being punctual. In this scenario, "being on time" falls within the domain of needs that have to do with Control and our Sense of Agency. To resolve this situation fully, the remaining step here would be to seek appropriate ways to meet the need, to gain the sense of control over when I am arriving at my destination. We talk more about this step in the next chapter (Step Three: Resource Awareness).

So to reiterate and to simplify, our inquiry into what we need looks like this:

- First, we ask — What am I feeling? This makes us aware of a negative emotion and alerts us to an unmet need.

- Next, we ask — What's wrong? This question validates that something isn't right *for us*, as opposed to something is wrong *with us*.

- Then, we ask — What makes it so? This question acknowledges that there was a reasonable trigger in the environment. (As I mentioned in Chapter 4, it is OK — and actually quite helpful — to ask what people/places/things made us feel a certain way, because it helps us understand what in our environment shifted and how that might have impacted our internal balance, as well as, which of our needs may now require attention because of that.)

- And finally, we ask — How does this [trigger] affect me? What's important to me? (This question is now specifically tapping into our needs and allows us to find out what needs are impacted, so that we can properly attend to them.)

The first three questions here are really Acknowledgment & Validation questions. They address our "emotional needs" (yes, I still do not like this term and this is the only time I will use it). Questions that seek to acknowledge and validate work like a good hug, when done right. The only right way to do that, by the way, is to do it without any judgment, be it around the emotion, the trigger, or the need. They soften the situation and make it OK to feel what we feel.

This acknowledgment and validation is necessary in order for us to move into the final steps of finding what needs are impacted. This would be impossible to do without the acknowledgment and validation. If we do not acknowledge and validate ourselves first about our feelings and experience, it will be impossible to feel seen and to truly understand what is at stake for us personally. By validating our feelings, we also validate our needs. And once we validate our needs, we can then focus on meeting them.

Here are additional ways to ask questions, as we engage in the "What's Wrong" inquiry:

- What is not working?
- What needs fixing?
- What is falling apart (or appears to be falling apart)?
- What needs to be attended to?

- What is asking for my attention?
- What is needed?
- What am I needing?
- What matters to me here?
- What do I want?

Note, however, that the answer to the last question cannot be an emotion. At least not the final answer. We can start there, but in order to get to a complete answer, we have to arrive at a need.

So if we say, "I want to feel good" or "I don't want to feel anxious" — that's alright as a starting point. But we must continue to find the need behind that emotion in order to resolve that emotion. And so we must also ask "What do I need in order to feel good and not feel anxious?" Another way of saying it is: "What is needed in order to feel good?" Asking these questions, sometimes repeatedly and with patience, can help point to the needs that are unmet or compromised. They will point to the area of need that requires our attention and us taking action, in order to meet the need through appropriate resources.

Although absolutely not required, we could get more nuanced with this process if we want to. And if we know which of the emotions in the Basic Triad we are working with, we can ask questions specific to that emotion, like this:

ANGER	SADNESS	FEAR
What is unjust or unfair? What am I called to protect, fix, or correct? What has been taken from me? What do I want to reclaim, or get back?	What am I losing? What am I missing? What am I wanting? What is meaningful/important? What's painful? What's hurting?	What is the threat? What am I concerned about? What do I not want to happen? What is at stake here? What am I likely to lose? What do I want to avoid?

It can also be as simple as restating the emotion in the following sentence: *What is this _______ all about?* Like this: "What is this *anger* all about?" We can also phrase it as: "What am I so *angry* about?" Just be careful not to sound judgmental or exasperated with yourself.

Answers to these questions will not only clearly point out the trigger, but also what was touched by the trigger and shifted out of balance for us. Now, we are not doing this to "blame" the trigger for our emotion, though that trigger is justifiably the cause of it. Doing this would be a waste of time. And so instead of that, we look into what we *need to do* about the situation to bring things back in-balance. What is it that we need to do, what actions can we take, to make sure our needs are met?

For example, we may be frustrated that a co-worker is stopping by to chat with us too often. Frustration is a feeling within the Anger continuum (see Appendix A for reference), and so if we ask the questions from this category, our answers may sound something like this:

What is unfair or unjust?

Answer: *Too many interruptions, I have a right to a quiet workplace.*

What needs to be protected or corrected?

Answer: *My time needs to be protected.*

What has been taken from me?

Answer: *My ability to do my work.*

What am I trying to get back?

Answer: *My focus, my time, a quiet place to work.*

In asking a series of questions, prompted by frustration (which is a form of anger), we are able to find out that the problem with this situation is that it is compromising our ability to focus and get our work done. And what we are discovering is that we need a proper environment to be productive. Although it is not necessary to identify which of the 8 Core Psychological Needs this belongs to in order for us to get our needs met, you may be curious to hear that this part depends on the particular individual who is experiencing this situation. For one person, the ability to focus, be productive, and manage their time will fall within the need for Agency & Control. Yet for another, it may be an expression of the need for Worth & Acknowledgment, if the project they are working on has to do with a big promotion they are after.

There is no wrong way to "label" the need, because each situation will express a different side of a Core Need for a particular person at a particular time. And finding a proper category is not the point.

Just like it is never the point of Step One to label an emotion "appropriately" (but rather to notice that it signals something important about our needs), same is true when it comes to need awareness. In this second step, we must place emphasis on understanding what is implicated, as opposed to what it is called. The 8 Core Psychological Needs discussed earlier and the labels associated with them are presented here so that you have a sense of your psychological world and the landscape of your psyche when you explore your needs. It's there to help you become more aware of your complex interior. It is intended to help you orient yourself, rather than test you on the knowledge of labels. Remember, we agreed to keep this simple and straightforward.

So let's return to our example. What do we do here? How do we meet our needs? We could blame our co-worker. Afterall, she is the one interfering with our needs. But that will not move us towards a solution. When we assign blame, we assign responsibility. And the one thing we must keep in mind is that we are the only ones that hold responsibility for our needs. Some people may be oblivious to the needs of others. Some may misinterpret our needs (in this case, a co-worker may be thinking we are looking forward to chatting any time, because we have been so willing and friendly thus far). Still others may simply be unhappy people themselves, who are attempting to meet their own needs at the expense of others.

I am not saying this to give us permission to judge others. I am saying this to point out that there is no way to know what may be going on for others, and it is much more productive to explore what is going on for us, and then take care of it ourselves. And so it is our job to respond to the trigger in a manner that meets our needs, as opposed to "attacking" the trigger. What we have to focus on is getting to the actual solution, where our needs can be met. So once we understand *what* we need by following the "What's Wrong" inquiry process (in our example it is the quiet space, protected time, etc.), we can decide on the action we want to take. And that is Step Three, which we explore in the next chapter.

* * *

One final thought on the "What's Wrong" inquiry before we move on. This is a bit of an advanced point, and so if it doesn't make sense right away, that's OK. When you practice the whole process over time, you will gain this insight naturally on your own, so do not worry. And that point is this: emotions can arise from the needs of both types, the needs of the Body (physical) and the needs of the Self (psychological). Typically, the needs of the body are communicated to us directly through sensations associated with the body (sensation of hunger or thirst, or muscle ache, etc.). But when they are neglected or not addressed, they tend to get compounded by an additional layer of signals in the form of emotions. This emotional signature amplifies the needs of the body to make sure we are paying attention to the original sensation that came from a physical need.

Let's look at some quick examples. We may feel anxious because we are concerned whether we will get enough sleep before a big event, or whether we will have a minute to run into the bathroom before catching the train, and so on. In these examples the needs we have to attend to are the needs of the body.

However, feeling tired, distracted, stressed, etc. can be an indication of either type of need. Meaning, we can be distracted because we are hungry and need to go eat something (a physical need), but it could also be because we are thinking about our favorite book (which speaks to the need for fun and enjoyment). Likewise, feeling tired can come from boredom and lack of stimulation, which is a reflection of a psychological need. But it can also be a reflection of a physical need from lack of proper sleep and our body's need for rest. Everything depends on the individual, because how our needs manifest themselves is dependent on who we are and what is going on for us in that moment.

How do *you* know which is which *for you*?

It comes from *knowing yourself*.

That self-knowledge will come over time from the practice of paying attention to ourselves. The best time to pay attention is when emotions arise and naturally call on us to pay attention to them. And then simply follow the 3-Step Needs-Based Process we have been discussing in this book:

Step 1 ⇒ Emotion Awareness (What are you feeling?)

Step 2 ⇒ Need Awareness (What do you need?)

Step 3 ⇒ Resource Awareness (What should you do about it?)

NEEDS VS. WANTS

Seeing how complex our needs are, we may be inclined to think that meeting them is a very complicated process. Not so. If this were the case, our needs would not be called basic and our wellbeing would not be dependent on them, because it would go against natural principles of evolution. In other words, complexity is only present when it serves an organism, not when it doesn't. Meeting our needs is much easier than we think and it should not tax our own internal system. The reason why it may seem difficult at first is because of our lack of understanding of what they are and how they show up in our own life.

Since these needs are core to who we are as human beings and are an expression of who we are as individuals, we are fully capable of finding resources to meet them (more on that in the next chapter). However, what *does* drain us and what *can* create a sense of burden is trying to fulfill every fleeting desire. Responding to every wish, want, and whim we may have — that is an enormous task and a huge drain on our resources. What becomes important is to learn to tell the difference between a core need and a "want," which is an expression of preference.

When it comes to meeting our needs, be it physical or psychological, it is never a question.

The answer is always a yes.

We have to find a way to meet them.

And there is always a way to meet our core needs because they are fundamental. How these needs are met will depend on the kind of resources available to us, but they always take priority over wants and wishes. When resources are plenty, we may have options and choices and can even meet several of our preferences that go beyond meeting our basic needs. However, when resources are limited, we make our *needs* a priority, while setting limits on the *wants* and the *preferences*. This makes it so that we make sure our needs are always met, which is the basis of feeling balanced, grounded, and content.

We do have the ability and the potential to meet our needs, as long as we understand what they are. Even if resources are limited and even if currently we may not feel like we have what is required to meet that need, we can still find a way (however imperfect), as long as we take responsibility for it and make it a priority. When we have a true need (as opposed to a want), we will mobilize to get resources. We will do what it takes to fulfill that need. If we'd rather not and prefer to do something else instead, or if we feel too lazy to go find resources — then what we are dealing with here is not a need, but a want.

Needs are non-negotiable, whereas wants — are.

But let's be clear: a want is not a bad thing at all. We all have preferences, and given a choice, would choose according to our preference. But when choices are not available or when resources are limited, we must prioritize getting needs met over insisting that our wants are satisfied instead. Wants are negotiable, but our needs are not. When we try to negotiate out of our needs, we deplete ourselves and risk living a life that is out of balance, unfulfilling, and even painful.

So how can you tell a want apart from a need?

Perhaps the simplest way to start is to look at this from the perspective of physical needs. When we feel hungry, that is a signal of a basic need for food. We respond to that need by eating *something*. If we have a choice of what to eat (meaning, our resources are plentiful), we may choose something that is more *desirable* and is in alignment with our *preference*. When we only have *one option* (say, the non-prefered leftovers), we will go for that to satisfy our need, even when it is not our preference.

However, if we insist that we've got to have more choices than the unappealing leftovers, then what we are doing at that moment is trying to indulge a *preference*, a *want*, not a need. This isn't a problem when we have options, but it becomes an issue when we don't. If we are truly hungry, we will make do with limited resources. Needs are not fussy. If we truly need food, we will satisfy it with what's available. But if we want a specific thing and will not eat unless we get that specific thing, then we are making things more difficult for ourselves. Or it simply means, we do not have a real need, and can wait. However, if it is a legitimate need and if this is something we do on a regular basis — argue with the reality of what is available to us — we either end up neglecting our needs or we end up wasting a lot of time and energy trying to accommodate a preference, not a necessity.

When it is truly *not* about a need, but rather we just *want* a specific thing, in that case we will have to be able to wait until that specific thing becomes available. That is also just fine, as long as we don't become obsessed and misinterpret that preference for a need that it isn't. This may sound counterintuitive at first, since our preferences can be so strong and we may be so stubborn about them that it can feel as though this must be a *need* talking, when in fact the opposite is true. The fussier we become about what we *want*, the less likely it is that we are dealing with a *need*. Our needs are so important, that when resources are limited, you will notice a natural tendency to accept the next best option.

When we are acting like we have choices, then we are clearly trying to satisfy a preference. If that is easy — great! But if we are stuck because we are fussy about our preferences, let's not confuse them for needs. It's not the needs that make us stuck, it is the wants that can get in the way of meeting our needs.

Let's look at another example and see how the need vs. the want dynamic may play out with a child. Now, even though we are using a child scenario as an example, it is relevant to everyone. I invite you to pay attention because often we too, act in a similar way when we have a limited perspective.

A child, just like a person of any age, has to satisfy their needs for curiosity and enjoyment. These are natural human needs that have to be honored to ensure proper development and a balanced psychological functioning. So parents typically make sure that this need is met by making time for that in the child's day, by creating space where they can play and explore. But when the child is insisting that the only fun thing in their life is a brand new toy, then they are speaking from a place of a want. When this want is declined, if the child has a true need for fun at that moment, they will move on and find something else to entertain themselves with. This happens naturally, because it is in our human nature to be on the lookout for alternative resources, when the ones we prefer are not available.

As I mentioned, *a want* can often masquerade as *a need* because it can sound as non-negotiable and demanding ("I will only be OK with *this*," or "This is the *only* way I will be happy"). In the case of the child from the previous example, upon hearing "No, we are not getting a new toy" the child may throw a tantrum and demand the toy even louder. That does not mean they have a *need* for a new toy, but rather they are expressing their disappointment at the fact that things are not going their way. If the child keeps insisting on this one thing, they will keep bumping against a "No" again and again, which delays meeting their actual need for fun.

The more specific the request, the more of a clue it is that this is a want, not a need. As soon as the child stops insisting that there is "only one way," many other options appear as to how to satisfy their need for fun and enjoyment. This is so because needs are actually quite flexible and not so demanding. The reason for that is because what's more important for our wellbeing is that they *are* met, not *how* they are met. From that angle, needs are easier to meet by finding an appropriate compromise to our preferences.

Now, children are young and may not always have the capacity to understand what is available to them and will benefit from help in finding compromises to meet their needs. This is where adults can support the child's ability to develop the skill of resourcefulness. However, as I mentioned, I bring up this example with a toy, because many adults seem to act this way too, getting stubborn about their wishes, and miss the opportunity to meet their needs by looking for alternative resources and ways to meet them.

For example, you may find yourself feeling bored, which is an expression of the need for Fun & Enjoyment. You may be thinking that getting together with a friend would be just the thing to do to meet that need. Turns out your friend is not available. OK, you are staying flexible and looking for other ways to meet the need by exploring what other enjoyable things you can do. You may decide to call another friend. And then another.

If no friends of yours are available and you are still focused on meeting your need of finding something enjoyable to do, as opposed to focusing on your specific preference (spending time with a friend), you will stay flexible. You will continue looking until you find something that satisfies that need, as opposed to pouting and getting upset that your friends are not available. If we were to do that, we would miss the opportunity to meet the need. Can you see that? When we are too busy pouting over a lack of preferred options, we stop looking at other resources, which in this case could be any other number of things that we would find enjoyable or fun.

If, however, nothing is fun or enjoyable and you can only think of spending time with friends as the way to meeting your need for fun & enjoyment then, my dear reader, the problem is not with your needs. The issue lies in lack of flexibility, which comes from your limited view of resources available to you. In this hypothetical scenario, what this means is that you have to expand your capacity and see more ways of meeting this need than how you have been doing it so far.

We talk more about building capacity in Chapter 8. But before we get there, let's take a look at resources in general and how we go about meeting our needs, which is Step Three in the 3-Step Needs-Based Process for handling emotions.

Chapter 6

Step Three: Resource Awareness

Living a full and *fulfilling life* requires you to use your resources. Why? Because resources help us satisfy our needs. There are resources all around us. Sometimes we don't see them because we may not be aware of them or may not be thinking of them as resources to tap into when we need something.

The fact that you have lived as long as you have and have had as many joys as you have, speaks to your ability to access resources. So we know you can do it, we just want to make sure you are doing it intentionally and on demand (when you have a need to take care of).

Without resources we perish.

Since you are reading this book, my hunch is you are far from that stage, which is very good news. (And if I guessed wrong, please put this book down and seek personalized support.) What would make your life even better is being aware of resources available to you, investing in new ones, and always being intentional about how you use what you have. Meaning, our resources should go towards meeting our needs, as opposed to being underutilized or even wasted.

As we discussed in the previous chapter, in addition to physical needs, we have 8 Core Psychological Needs that encompass other more nuanced expressions of what we may be seeking or needing. We also discussed how important it is to attend to the full spectrum of our needs on a regular basis. Since these universal core needs are expressed in unique and individual ways, how they are met will differ from one person to another, and so each one of us will have to find what works for us personally. Consequently, as we will discuss in this chapter, we have to become aware of what resources are available specifically to us and which of those resources work for us the best when it comes to meeting our individual needs.

For example, one person may seek a greater connection within themselves, while another may feel a need to connect more with peers. One person will need a lot of social interactions, while another — very little. I may find enjoyment in being in nature, while someone else finds the answer in playing a musical instrument. There are so many answers to our needs, but finding what works for you and your unique make up is what matters most. Simply doing what other people do is not what will give us fulfillment, and will leave our needs unmet. We can certainly get ideas from others and how they go about accessing resources, but we always have to test whether that works for us personally.

The goal is to stay active in searching for the right answers to the needs that our emotions pointed to. Staying actively engaged in this process is what makes us responsive to our needs and, therefore, more likely to satisfy them. So let's talk about that.

FROM EMOTION TO ACTION

To begin, let's revisit the example of a chatty coworker, which we discussed in the previous chapter. The actions we ultimately take here, to resolve this situation and meet our needs, will depend on what resources we have available to us and what else we are able and willing to explore.

For example, if our relationship with the co-worker is a good one — that is a resource. We can use this resource (i.e., good relationship) to talk to her about our preferences in a way that she would understand and respect. If we have good communication skills — that is also a resource. We can gently but firmly articulate our boundaries even to those with whom we don't have close relationships. If we have another location to work from, a door with a lock, and a "do not disturb" sign — all of these are resources too. We can choose to utilize them or look for other ones based on what we think will work best for us.

Which of these resources we go for first depends on our assessment of which one is easier to implement and which one is more likely to result in the outcome we want. In this case, the need we are looking to meet is to have conditions that allow us to focus and have uninterrupted work time.

These are examples of thoughtful approaches to meeting a need.

It takes not only having awareness and understanding of our needs, but also some practice in finding *appropriate* ways to do so. There is no judgment around the fact that initially we may be compelled to respond to an emotion in impulsive or reactive ways. Nor is there a judgment about the fact that we don't always choose to act in ways that serve us. That happens. We are all learning, and we all make mistakes. Rest assured, this will change with time. As we become more aware of resources available to us, we will be able to pick more effectively what works for us best.

The stronger our emotions, the more compelled we feel to react. To avoid spontaneous blow-ups and impulsive reactions we may later regret, it helps if we notice our emotions early on. When they show up in the form of less intense nudges, we can take the opportunity to respond to the needs they signal about in a proactive manner. And so, if we think about our scenario, let's not wait until we have missed several deadlines, before we decide to do something about our chatty coworker. Because if we do it then, it is not likely to go well, since — having been deprived of uninterrupted work time — we are less likely to show up calmly and resolve the situation appropriately.

The purpose of our emotions is not just to *communicate* our needs to us. That is only the first part of it. The second and the most important reason we have emotions is — *to act.* Let's revisit this diagram from Chapter 2:

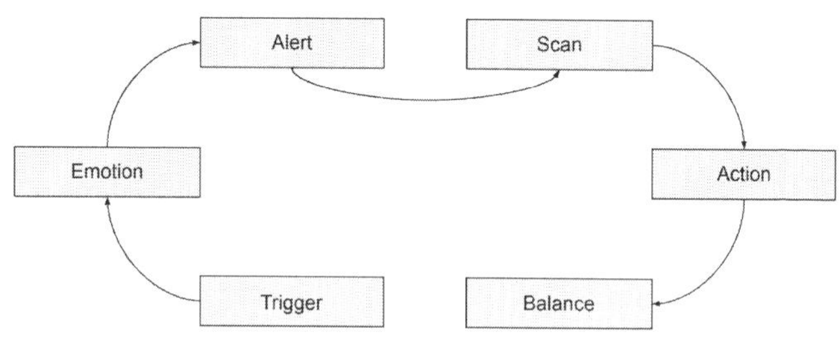

From this perspective, emotions are designed *to move us* into action, to do something in order to meet the needs we have. You may have heard people say that "emotion is just energy, energy in motion" (as in *e*-motion, where "e" stands for *e*nergy). I consider this phrase gimmicky and not practical. It suggests that we must interpret this "energy in motion" as something that comes and goes, as something that flows in and out of you... as if it's not yours to claim, or not related to you. As if it is something you just happened to come by. Like the wind — you just happened to be in its way and you just wait for it to pass by and around you.

Now, don't get me wrong, emotions *are* energy, and we do feel them as energetic manifestations, as either positively or negatively charged. But they are not random, impersonal, and unrelated to us. In other words, the energy of emotions is not just "flowing in and out," nor is it chaotic.

It is both *directional* and *intentional.*

It directs you to act.

Act with an intention to meet your needs.

If we are to talk about motion and movement as it relates to emotions, here is a critical element many people miss. It isn't the emotion that has to move. It isn't the energy of that emotion either. What has to move is *the person* having the emotion. You and I, when we experience unpleasant emotions, must move to take action.

The essential purpose of emotions is to set *us* in-motion.

They move us, they compel us *to get in-to-motion, to take action.* Emotions are the energy that comes up and prompts: do, go, act, seek, respond, find a way. The higher the need and the more intense the emotion, the more *moved and pulled* into action we feel.

The problem is that we misinterpret this surge of energy as a bad thing and do everything we can to hold back. So instead of moving into an appropriate action to meet the need behind this emotion, we try to "contain" it, squash it down, ignore it, or we decide to just sit-with-it to "let emotions pass."

In doing any of that, we are missing the point. You can see how counterproductive that is to the actual purpose, which is — to move towards meeting our needs.

Sometimes the actions and the doing, required to meet the needs, are minor and sometimes it takes quite a bit of effort. But those actions do have to be intentional and start with an inquiry as to what we are feeling and what may be needed: what has to be attended to and what has to be responded to. These are the things we discussed in the previous chapter within the "What's Wrong" inquiry section.

At the same time, this activating power of emotion is also the reason why so many people may act impulsively when driven by feelings, because emotions — especially at higher levels of intensity — are quite forceful in their energy. Emotions are drives. They contain motivating energy, whether the charge they carry is negative or positive, the outcome emotions "seek" is functional and adaptive. And that is — to transform themselves into the *energy of action* that takes care of whatever is required to be taken care of.

Emotions, be they big or small, fuel our actions.

They move us *forward*.

They compel us *to act.*

They are not for sitting on or sitting with (only insofar as we need to comprehend what we are feeling and why). In fact, if we only sit and do not take action supported by our emotions, we may miss out on that extra energy, drive, and motivation to do what needs to be done. I am not speaking about impulsive action, but rather about the determination, conviction, and pull to take the action that our emotions come with and that will get us closer to meeting our needs.

And that action does not have to be impulsive. It can be measured, deliberate, thoughtful, and considerate of our resources. If we let emotions "flow in and out" (which isn't how it works anyway), we are missing out on the energetic resource that comes with our emotions. If we ignore it or try to squash it down, we create an environment of misdirected energy that expresses itself in unexpected, unintentional, and — quite impulsive ways.

Trapped emotions are actually trapped *action energy*. Meaning it is the action potential that did not materialize.

When we check in with our emotions and understand our needs, the answer as far as what action to take may not always be the answer we like. Let's be honest, sometimes we may prefer to be grouchy and pout at other people instead of focusing our efforts on meeting our needs. An intense feeling of anger, for example, does not direct us to punch a wall, but it does tell us that things have gone too far and an appropriate action is required from us to resolve the source of distress.

If you are not used to actively looking for resources to meet your needs, you will find yourself more prone to impulsivity (such as acts of aggression when angry). You may also find it easier to blame others, because then you do not feel the responsibility to take action. You pass it on to others. But ultimately, it is through taking action and feeling compelled to take care of ourselves and our needs that we come to appreciate the kind of power and strength that comes from satisfying personal needs. This sense of being in-balance and having our needs met can never come from pouting and waiting on others to pay attention to us and to serve us. Seeing the responsibility in ourselves to attend to our own needs is empowering in a very genuine, rich, and meaningful way.

It is the kind of strength that gives us back control over our lives, makes our cup full, and supports our sense of vitality and aliveness.

When through our own actions we are validated time and time again, when our emotions are seen as real, true, and valuable, when our needs are met, all of that — deeply affirms who we are. That deep sense of affirmation supports our sense of Self, builds strength, confidence, and self-esteem. Now, think about this... How different this feels compared to what is generally called "thoughtwork," a process where the message we tell ourselves sounds something like "my brain is the problem" or "there is nothing wrong with the environment, there is something wrong with me and my thoughts."

How invalidating and how far from the truth!

If we are responding to something with emotions, that only means that there is a prompt, a trigger in the environment, the world around us. The only difference is that we are not asking our environment to fix it for us. We are looking to ourselves, to our resources, to our skills, and to our capacity to find solutions.

So let's build our awareness around resources.

HAVING ACCESS TO RESOURCES

When we respond to emotions, the purpose of our actions is to find a resource that matches our need. When that does not happen, we end up with unmet needs (which is something we discuss in more detail in the next chapter). And as I like to say, your needs are not your problem, the problem is your *unmet needs*. In other words, the problem is not that we have them, but that we ignore them.

How do we end up ignoring our needs?

First, by ignoring emotions.

Then, by failing to identify the need.

And finally, by failing to act.

The reason we take action is so that our needs are met. Taking action requires understanding what resources are available to us to satisfy our needs. Of course, this also presumes that we have an understanding of what specific need we are trying to satisfy. And we also have to be mindful not only about taking action but also about *continuing to take action* until the need is met.

Let me repeat this again. It is not enough to act. We must act *until* the need is met, because the whole point of taking action is to meet the need. So if we tried talking to a co-worker and it didn't resolve the issue of constant interruptions, we have to do something else.

In order to access resources to meet our needs, we have to be aware that those resources exist in the first place. In other words, we must understand that there are many ways to satisfy our needs. Not only that, but that there is *always* a way to meet our needs. If we find it challenging, it is either because we do not have clarity around our needs or we may be nit-picky about a preference and are hyperfocused on options not available to us at the moment. Once we are generally aware of what kind of resources tend to meet *our* needs, we can be proactive about having access to those resources and to the things that tend to work for us.

In order to begin to cultivate awareness of resources we have to, first and foremost, understand that it is our own responsibility to look after ourselves and our needs. Although it is our environment that in many ways impacts how we feel and triggers an emotional response, it isn't the environment that is ultimately responsible for why we continue to feel bad or why our wellbeing worsens. So, what is it then? It is our failure to respond in a proper way to what is happening. In other words, we don't feel bad because of our environment per se. We feel bad because we do not do anything about it. Life, environment, other people, etc. — they show us where our needs are and we must understand that there is something we have to do about our needs in order to meet them.

Where we place the responsibility is where we place our dependence.

Meaning, if we expect others, the environment, the situation, etc. to change, then we will be dependent on those people, places, and things. Sometimes it so happens that the conditions in our environment change in our favor without us doing anything and that's great. Say, the chatty coworker got moved to a different department, and we can now work without interruptions. However, most of the time what others decide to do or not to do is not in our control.

It is so much wiser, then, to lean on our own Sense of Agency and rely on ourselves. Besides, it is important that we understand what it is *we can do* to meet our needs and not confuse that with what happened fortuitously. Happy accidents — like a coworker being moved to another department — cannot be considered our own resource. Meaning, this is not something we can rely on in the future and will not be able to meet our needs this way should someone else become a distraction.

As was previously mentioned, despite the fact that needs are universal and all humans have them, the way they are expressed and fulfilled is very individual. Because of that, the kind of resources we seek and are able to access is also very individual. Some resources are simple and some more advanced, some are obtained through other people and some are accessed on our own.

Our ultimate goal is to move away from being dependent on other people in meeting our needs towards being able to meet our needs independently of others. And so growing our capacity to access resources we can rely on (i.e., being resourceful) is critical to our ability to have our needs met on a regular basis and to feeling taken care of.

Growing our own internal resources through personal development and cultivation of additional skills and abilities can also help us with that tremendously. This way, when we find ourselves in situations where resources may be generally limited, we have internal reserves to tap into. For example, you may not have thought of it but the need for Connection & Belonging can be met not only through connection with other people, but also through cultivating a deep connection with ourselves, or with what we may call — the Higher Power, Spirit, God, The Universe, Life Source, etc. — all of which are examples of internal resources.

Our typical definition of resources is rather limited.

It can limit what we perceive as a resource.

Usually what people mean when they talk about resources are things like money, time, connections, and things (all the "stuff" in our lives). Although, undeniably, these are great, there is so much more to resources than that! The more open we are to finding ways of meeting our needs, the more resources we will find. Resourcefulness requires flexibility and open mindedness.

Conversely, the more fixated we are on insisting we meet our needs a certain way and only in that way, the more narrow our options become. In that case, we have to be willing to tolerate that scarcity. At the same time, we have to be mindful not to sacrifice our needs for the sake of meeting a want, a trivial preference, as this will only be of disservice to us (something we discussed in the Needs vs. Wants section of the previous chapter). Our wellbeing depends on the satisfaction of our needs, and not on pleasing every whim or approving every impulse. A genuine need most always has a way of being satisfied, even when resources are limited due to the conditions of a specific situation. As long as we don't eliminate potential resources by our own insistence on particular preferences, we are going to do alright.

Now, I don't want there to be a misunderstanding. I am not saying that preferences are not important. Preferences, wants, and desires do have their own time and place — which is usually when we have choices and our resources are plentiful. At all other times, we have to focus on the underlying needs first, and be mindful that we are not creating unnecessary tension of unmet needs due to our own capriciousness.

TAKE INVENTORY OF YOUR RESOURCES

So what kind of resources are we talking about? There are resources we already possess but may not recognize as such. And there are other resources out there that we don't yet have or that we may not have considered, but that can give us more options when tapped into. This section is intended to help you see some of the things that can help you meet your needs. This is not an exhaustive review (a whole separate book would be needed to do that!), and so in this section I want to provide you with a starting point and, hopefully, it will give you ideas to explore even further.

Positive Emotions

To begin with, let's consider positive emotions. You may not have thought of it, but positive emotions provide us with many clues as to where our resources may be. This is because positive emotions signal satisfied needs. Having satisfied needs means there were resources — or ways — which helped in meeting those needs.

Most of us miss out on this resource, because we usually don't think much about our positive emotions. Typically these are not the feelings people tend to struggle with and because of that, we don't pay much attention to them. Generally, these emotions tell us "all is well." And so it would be really helpful for you to notice what happens during those times that makes you feel that all is well, that your needs are met and things are in-balance.

When you pay attention to these things, you can start noticing what happened prior to your needs being met and then use this knowledge to recreate those opportunities for yourself again in similar situations. For example, if you know having good relationships with your coworkers becomes a reliable resource you can tap into when tension arises in the workplace, then you can proactively invest in developing solid mutually respectful connections at work.

To tap into this area of resources we need to explore what is already working and ask what makes it so? What makes you feel good? How can you have more of that in your life?

One thing we have to be mindful of here is the following: there is a difference between positive emotions that are generated through *distraction* and positive emotions that come from a *satisfied* need. How can you tell the difference? When we feel emotional discomfort or distress and find a distraction that takes our mind off of it, we will feel positive emotions. However, they are fleeting. If, as soon as that thing, the distraction, is stopped, you feel down — that's a clear sign that you were avoiding another negative emotion and did not address the actual need underneath it.

Distractions are not good resources.

A true resource that meets a need will result in sustained positive emotion. Those are the areas we want to explore, not the ones that generate fleeting positive emotions and only serve as a distraction from discomfort. For example, if music makes you happy, but you feel down as soon as it stops, then music is not meeting your needs at that moment. What it does, though, is it helps you distract yourself from discomfort that some unmet need has created. Maybe you were listening to music to "drown" your feelings about how your day at work went. You'd need to reflect about what needs were implicated and look for other solutions, other ways, and other resources to address what's not working. Likewise, if you feel energized around happy people, but feel low as soon as they are gone, something is not right. The fact that your positive emotions did not last means that the social interaction was rather superficial or irrelevant to what is really going on, and was not a match for your needs.

Skills, Knowledge & Experience

Depending on the situation, it may be specific knowledge or a skill that will help you meet your needs. Also, having experience meeting a need successfully, will make taking care of it next time that much easier. This is your knowledge of yourself at work and it is an asset to you. You won't have to think too long to be able to tell what works for you in which situations because of that acquired wisdom of self-knowledge. With that in mind, apply this perspective to the area of needs you are still trying to figure out. In other words, know that meeting your needs gets easier over time, because you gain a better understanding of yourself through experience.

Other people's knowledge, skills, and tools can also be of resource to you. You can benefit from them when you cannot do something yourself or, even if you can, you prefer not to for whatever reason (such as, for example, preserving your resources). For example, you *could* paint your house yourself, but may you prefer not to. Or, say, you *could* learn how to fix your car by finding someone to teach you, but you may want a mechanic to do it for you instead.

Obviously, these are exaggerated and simplistic examples, and that is on purpose, because they are meant to illustrate a point. In your life, however, you will find similar but different and more nuanced examples of where you may need to either build your own resource of skills and knowledge, or find others who already have them. It all comes down to how you prefer to manage your resources and what makes the most sense for you.

One thing to understand, though, is that when it comes to psychological needs, it is our responsibility to meet them. This is not something we can delegate to others, even when we ask for help.

Whereas someone can fix leaking pipes in our house, when we are dealing with "leaks" in our emotional world, this is something we will have to learn to do on our own. This does not mean that you *learn this by yourself* — there is definitely a lot of good guidance out there and professional help — but that you learn to be able to *apply this on your own*. Speaking of leaks, let's talk about our energy reserves and our energy capacity.

Energy Reserves

One of the ways we feel resourceful is when we have *high levels* of energy. Have you ever thought about where our energy and the sense of vitality comes from? Why do we feel fluctuations in our energy? Our energy levels have *everything* to do with our needs. Satisfied needs result in having more energy and a higher sense of aliveness. Sometimes satisfying one type of needs will generate energy that helps meet other types of needs. For example, physical energy can help us find resources that meet our psychological needs. Likewise, having mental capacities and an overall balanced sense of psychological wellbeing can help us problem-solve around the best way to meet our physical needs.

Regularly satisfied needs equal *stable levels* of energy. When we are well-balanced and most of our needs are met, we have a more reliable flow of energy. However, when we are overwhelmed and dealing with too many competing priorities and are neglecting most of our needs — we have less energy and, when it comes, it is unpredictable. Sometimes we deplete ourselves so much, we cannot even see resources available to us to get ourselves out of that depleted state.

If you are concerned about a potential conundrum of needing to have energy in order to create it (or if you are asking yourself, "But how do I meet my needs if I have no energy for it?"), don't worry. We typically do not ignore *all* of our needs at *all* times. This would mean our energy reserves are at complete zero. If this were the case, you would not be reading a book right now. What is more true is that most of the time at least *some* of our needs are met, and so we can use that minimum of energy and attend to a few more of our needs.

- The more needs we meet, the more of them we become able to meet.

This is because our energy increases with each need we attend to. We just want to make sure we don't *waste* energy on pursuits that do not meet our needs. This is also why, by the way, dealing with emotions the traditional way can feel depleting. For example, blaming our brain for our thoughts is not going to meet our needs, but it is quite energy consuming and so, instead of giving us energy, it takes it away. It is important to understand that we *always* exert energy when we are engaged with the world, when pursuing our goals, and meeting our needs. However, *using* energy is different from *wasting* it.

We can drive a car and use gas to get us somewhere, or we can idle in park-mode, go nowhere, and waste gas. In either case, gas gets depleted. And so since we always use energy, we want to make sure we use it productively. Not to mention, we also have to make sure we refill our reserves regularly by continuing to attend to our needs.

You may have sensed that you have different kinds of energy.

Probably, the physical energy of our body is the one you are most immediately aware of. The energy in the body comes from satisfaction of physical needs. So when our body needs more energy, when we feel thirsty or hungry, we can sense this clearly, can get ourselves nourished, and bring our physical energy back to its optimal level. It may be the case that our body needs rest, and so then rest is how we increase our physical energy.

Some of us are also very aware of those moments in the day when our *mental* energy is diminishing. For example, we can notice that we are not as focused, our moment-to-moment memory is somewhat dull. We may be thinking, "Wait, what did I want to do next? Why did I open this file?" We may be noticing that our comprehension drifts and we find ourselves re-reading the same line over and over. All those things that make you feel like a fog is setting in... Can you relate?

Well, these are some of the signs of low mental capacity, and to get this type of energy back up we wouldn't be feeding ourselves another lunch or doing the kinds of things we would normally do to restore our physical energy. No. Instead, we may need to take a break, get some fresh air, switch to another task or activity that will engage us on a different level. We may change environments, add or eliminate background noise, and any number of things that *work for you*.

That is key.

Finding *what works for you* based on your needs and how you tend to meet them is vital. There are many different things we could do to restore energy. What *you* need to do is the thing that works *for you*. This applies to needs across the whole spectrum (physical and psychological). Finding resources for meeting our needs is not usually a problem. It is our *perspective* around our needs that may be at the root of our dissatisfaction. So let's spend a minute here next.

Personal Resources

The more awareness and understanding we have about our needs, the better able we are to find resources to meet them. And the better we get at finding the right resources, the more able we are to satisfy those needs without waiting for others to accommodate us. Some of the most critical resources you have access to are your own internal qualities, skills, and strengths. We can call them — personal resources.

These include things like: emotional balance (which comes from proactively meeting your needs), reasoning and problem-solving capacities, interpersonal qualities and relationships skills, personal attributes (such as resilience, perseverance, determination), strength (health and energy), sense of purpose, values, self-awareness, and so on. That's a lot of options! When some resources are low or inaccessible, other resources can be developed even more to compensate for the low areas. As I mentioned earlier, what you soon will find is that our own needs, when fulfilled, become a resource in and of itself and can help access additional resources. For example, when we are living a purposeful life and generally feel fulfilled, it is easier to problem-solve around challenges and see ways to resolve them.

Personal resources are those intangible qualities that make us who we are. They include our character, level of personal maturity, the degree of our self-awareness, and the way we think. Our mindset, things we tell ourselves, beliefs and perspectives we adopt, etc. — all of them shape how we see things. They either help us or prevent us from seeing opportunities and resources we have. Our thinking style is the way we tend to perceive things, assess our situation, evaluate options, and problem-solve in general.

Are we open minded and solution-oriented, or closed-off and problem-oriented?

Are we willing to ask for help when necessary, or do we insist on doing everything on our own?

How quickly do we give up and do we have resilience?

Having or not having these qualities and capacities does impact how well we are able to meet our needs. In Chapter 8, we dive deeper into this topic when we talk about building capacity for more. For now, I just want you to be aware that personal resources is a huge territory where we may find additional resources for meeting our needs.

Your ability to problem solve does not only depend on your world-view and perspective (such as, for example, believing that solutions are out there vs. believing you are doomed to suffer), but also on specific problem-solving skills. Sometimes, even with the best of perspectives and a great attitude, you still may need to know how to approach a particular situation. Here I am speaking about specific skills and knowledge, which may be required to resolve a particular need. And so, it also takes knowing the difference between an attitude problem vs. a knowledge/skill problem when looking for a proper resource.

- What we think of ourselves also has a lot to do with how we go about caring for ourselves.

Do we even allow the idea that we are worthy and that our needs have to be respected and attended to? Don't dismiss this question. Really think about it. One of the critical factors that play a role in being able to develop and access our own personal resources, is taking responsibility for our needs. When we understand that our needs are our responsibility, we get more engaged in figuring out how to meet them.

Maybe you are so tied up in taking care of other people that taking care of yourself seems to be a privilege, not a right, and definitely not a personal duty. Maybe you think that meeting our needs becomes impossible — or even unnecessary — when we become parents, face life challenges, take care of frail family members, manage huge teams at work, and so on. I feel you. And I get it. But what I invite you to see is that this is a belief, a perspective, and not a helpful one. You can challenge this perspective.

In fact, you can challenge *any* perspective that is not serving you.

How do you tell whether it's serving you? By the way it makes you feel. If it's not working, you will feel an ongoing presence of one or more feelings from the Triad of Discomfort (anger, sadness, or worry), and most likely — a lot of resentment too.

If you turned away from your own needs and crossed yourself out as someone insignificant, it is not because of your work, your children, or your ailing parents. It is because you have been introduced to and started believing a certain narrative of how your life should be when you take on new responsibilities — full of endless sacrifices.

But how true is that?

It is one way of thinking, for sure, but there is also a different one — the one that allows you to see your own humanity and embrace your needs as belonging to someone worthy and important. As a valuable person to yourself, you can be aware of your energy levels and do the best that you can at maintaining your own tank full.

NEED & RESOURCE MATCH

Accessing resources is not the only thing to keep in mind. Most importantly, we must make sure that we are using the right resources for the right needs. For example, from the perspective of the physical needs, we shouldn't be eating when we are thirsty. We should be drinking something. And we shouldn't be drinking something when we are tired. We should be resting. Our resource should match the need. Otherwise, the need will go unsatisfied and continue causing discomfort.

Earlier, we explored how satisfying some needs will generate energy that helps meet other needs. What is important to understand here is that we can only generate energy when we match needs with proper resources, because energy is generated only when a need is met in a proper way. In other words, physical strength comes from meeting physical needs, mental strength comes from meeting our mental needs, personal strength comes from meeting psychological needs, and so on. It is like putting the proper type of fuel for the kind of engine our car has.

When we confuse our needs, we may try to meet the needs of the Self with resources meant for our body. And just as a good meal will not take care of your psychological needs, only tending to psychological needs will not sustain your body. That's how we risk running into trouble, when we fail to meet our needs across the whole spectrum. That leads to dysfunctional outcomes. If we do this a lot, we begin to quietly — or not so quietly — suffer. No wonder why so many of us do not feel satisfied with our lives!

Some of us are so depleted that in our desperation we are doing anything and everything, which — contrary to our expectations — depletes us even more. It is what they call a throw-spaghetti-at-the-wall kind of strategy to see what sticks. Of course, it is more important to try *something* than to do nothing, when it comes to looking for the right match to our needs. So let's say that, even though I do not recommend it, I *reluctantly* approve of this strategy as a last resort.

However, what I am most concerned with is that when we "throw spaghetti at the wall" we rarely pause to look at what actually sticks. That gets in the way of us noticing what actually worked for us.

We need to be a little bit more aware of what we are doing and what we are getting out of it.

The importance of taking action when we have signs of discomfort or distress cannot be underestimated. The whole point of negative emotions is to drive action, to make us seek resources that will meet a need. The thing we don't want to end up doing, though, is acting impulsively because then it is more likely that we will end up with a need/resource mismatch.

Although our emotional reactions are spontaneous and automatic (nothing's wrong with that, as we saw in Chapter 2), our response to our needs should be thoughtful, mindful, and intentional as much as we can help it. Our goal is to match a resource to the need, which requires understanding that need to begin with, and that takes some reflecting upon and paying attention to. This is something you cannot do if you are going about your needs in a haphazard way. It is not very likely that we can hit a moving target with a blindfold on, is it? The only thing we would get out of that is an outcome we do not desire.

If that happens, however, we don't have to panic because when we are thoughtful and intentional, we can evaluate the outcomes to see whether what we did is meeting our needs or not, and whether it is actually creating additional challenges and problems. It's all part of the process.

We can always try again, and then again, and seek other more appropriate means and resources to meet those needs. At the same time, if aiming at a moving target, so to speak, with a blindfold on is — for whatever reason — your only option at the moment, then go for it, knowing that you would have to be willing to be patient and try several times.

What can I say? You might get lucky! And that, once again, is better than doing nothing. However, my point is:

- Luck is not a strategy
  when it comes to meeting our needs.

A better way to go about things is to get to know our needs more intentionally. It's a good practice to have — to observe ourselves and how we navigate the world, and take note of what works for us and what doesn't. You may be wondering, what is the best gauge for that? Our emotions, of course! How we feel about things tells us whether we are on the right track or not.

You may have heard that it is not a good idea to take action based on emotions. And that, especially when we feel a negative emotion, taking action from that place leads to negative outcomes and that we end up causing more problems. That is not true.

Let's consider the following: Anger can lead us to finally solving a challenge, or finally making things right. For example, when someone has been taking advantage of us, anger helps us to finally realize that enough is enough. Sadness can help us reflect on the loss of something we care about and truly appreciate its meaning. And from there it can prompt us to preserve and honor what matters. For example, say we realized we have wasted a whole day on social media and accomplished nothing of what we truly wanted. We feel disappointed (which is an emotion on the Sadness continuum) and so we can take steps to protect our time going forward.

These examples illustrate that negative emotions (i.e., emotions that carry a negative charge) can lead to positive outcomes, which contradicts the common misconception that negative emotions are inherently bad and lead to impulsive actions and negative outcomes. The difference in the examples offered is that — these were *thoughtful* actions. They were actions that matched the need, as opposed to impulsive actions that do not.

The only thing that determines whether we get a positive outcome or a negative one is whether the way we chose to go about meeting our needs actually resulted in those needs being met. When we understand our needs and know what is the best way to satisfy them, we have a need/resource match.

When needs are met, the outcome of our actions is *functional*. When there is a need/resource mismatch and the need is not met, the outcome is *non-functional,* or even *dys-functional*.

The simple way to differentiate between the two is to think of non-functional outcomes as *not getting what we wanted*, whereas dysfunctional outcomes are about *getting what we didn't want*. This happens when instead of meeting a need, we create more problems. For example, for those who eat cake (a perceived answer/resource) every time they are upset (note that several needs may be at play here), not only do they fail to resolve the need underneath that emotion, they are also gaining undesired weight. And so here we see both a non-functional outcome (i.e., not getting the need met) and a dysfunctional one (i.e., gaining weight).

To make it more likely that we have *functional* outcomes from our actions, we should seek to understand what actions would be the most appropriate. We do this based on our *emotion* and what we understand our *need* to be, instead of engaging in various self-soothing strategies or distractions that will inevitably lead to mismatch between the need and the resource.

Self-soothing is commonly suggested as a strategy for dealing with negative emotions. Although it may be a great *technique* to de-escalate strong emotions in the moment (so that we can actually think about resources available to us), on its own it is *not a strategy* for resolving emotions. Why? Because self-soothing does not address or resolve unmet needs. If you only engage in self-soothing activities and do nothing else, you will quickly find that it does not truly work, which shows you that it is not a resource, but rather a *tactic* to get you through the rough spot until you find appropriate resources. It is a bandaid.

Let's look at an example. If we get berated by our boss to the point where we have to hide in the bathroom to take deep breaths, or tell ourselves mantras and affirmations in order to face the world again, then we are not really solving the problem, are we? We may be feeling calmer and more composed after self-soothing, which can get us through that moment, but our work does not end here as we still have to take care of what is truly needed. You will know this to be true if you continue to self-soothe as soon as you get home from work. In an effort to "get over it" you may engage in additional self-soothing tactics and do things like calling a friend to vent about work, popping some wine to relax and "forget about it," binge watching movies until you fall asleep, and other things like that.

Now, don't get me wrong. If you are watching a movie because that has been your plan all along, you have been looking forward to it, and you really want to, then that is a match for your need for Enjoyment. If you are calling your friend because that is what you normally do, that's a match for your need for Connection. But in this case, if we were to do these things because of a rough day, do we *really* have a match for our needs? Are all these — and many more — self-soothing techniques providing a solution to what truly bothers us? No.

Let's take a closer look and ask, first of all, what need may be implicated in that scenario? The answer to that depends on who we are, what emotions we felt when berated by the boss (angry? sad? anxious?), as well as our unique expression of needs. (By the way, this may be a good place to remind you that all 8 Core Psychological Needs are listed in Appendix B, alongside a basic list of physical needs.)

If we felt intimidated or attacked in this example, our need may be safety. If we feel hurt and devalued, our need may be acknowledgment or respect. And so you can see how self-soothing techniques may help us through the day but do not actually address these needs. Although they can relieve the intensity of emotions and give you some space to breathe and calm down, it is not the answer.

Self-soothing may meet your "emotional needs" (see discussion in Chapter 5 and the difference between psychological needs and emotional needs), but it is not going to address the actual trigger and the psychological need involved. In order for that to happen, in addition to helping ourselves calm down, we also must take action to meet the underlying needs. So in this example, a better match to our needs would be navigating that toxic dynamic at work and setting proper boundaries. This is easier said than done, of course, especially if we do not have the skills or practice for handling similar situations. And sometimes it will require trying out several resources — from getting formal support at work, to using skills of assertiveness, to perhaps finding a better job environment for ourselves, among other things.

Ultimately, the way we will know we used the right resource is when we have our needs met. Whether the need we had in this scenario was the one for safety, respect, or acknowledgment, our actions have to match that need. The way to know whether the need is met, is if we no longer feel discomfort or distress about that situation and if it feels resolved. And this leads us to the final stage of the process, which is — evaluating outcomes. This is us checking in with ourselves, looking at the results of our actions, and assessing whether the need is satisfied or whether something else has to be tried in order to give ourselves what we need.

EVALUATING OUTCOMES

So we know it is important to find the proper means of satisfying our needs, but how do we know we did that? How do we tell whether there was a proper match and the need is appropriately met? Let's talk about it.

I think it is easier for us to tell when our *physical* needs are not met, because we are more in-tune with them, so let's start here. If we were hungry, ate a cracker, and are still hungry — it is pretty clear that a cracker isn't going to do it. The fact that we are still hungry shows that a cracker is not the proper resource match for our level of need, and that we have to get something more substantial. On the other hand, if a couple of crackers did the trick, great — looks like a small snack is all we needed. Likewise, when we wake up after 4 hours of sleep, it is pretty clear that we need more rest. However, if we feel refreshed after 20-30 minutes of sleep — great! Looks like we just needed a quick nap. That is how we assess the outcome of our actions and see whether there was a match between the need and the resources utilized.

Although it is easier to evaluate outcomes around physical needs, it may not always be as clear when it comes to our *psychological* needs. This is especially true if we are just learning to pay attention to them. And that is OK. Getting to know ourselves better is certainly a process. And we approach this process in the same way that we take care of our physical needs — we pay attention, we listen, and we check in to see if the actions we took did what we needed them to do.

What makes finding the right resources for our psychological needs a bit more of a guessing game, especially initially, is the fact that we start out not having full awareness of what these needs are to begin with. In order to detect our needs, we have to have knowledge about these 8 Core Psychological needs as their own separate — though certainly interconnected — areas of need. Meaning, just like we cannot resolve hunger by sleeping, thirst by exercising, and muscle aches by drinking soda, we cannot meet one psychological need through resources that are not meant for it.

In other words, we cannot meet our need for Meaning & Purpose by seeking attention from others. And while we meet our need for Fun & Enjoyment, we still have to make sure we have our need for Comfort & Safety fulfilled as well. Likewise, what is a good way to meet our need for Connection, may not be a good way of meeting our need for Autonomy or Control.

We will not get it right immediately.

And that is not a problem.

When we evaluate what outcome we got and ask ourselves, whether what we did addressed the need we had, we will be able to tell, whether the outcome was: functional (i.e., the need was met), non-functional (i.e., the need was *not* met), or dysfunctional (i.e., the need was not met *and* our actions created additional problems).

When we don't understand our 8 Core Psychological Needs as separate kinds of needs, we will get fewer hits than misses. It's part of the exploration process and we will eventually learn, as long as we are paying attention to what we are doing and the outcomes we are getting. Initially, we may end up trying strategies and doing things that worked for one need, but do not result in a desirable outcome when applied to another need.

This becomes very obvious when we try to resolve *psychological* needs with resources we use for *physical* needs. It may sound funny when I put it this way, but we do, in fact, do that. Why? Because meeting physical needs is often habitual and we tend to be good at it. Sometimes when we are good at something, we do it on autopilot, which is not always ideal.

For example, when we feel emotional discomfort or distress (both of which are signs of *psychological* needs) we may choose to eat, or take a nap, or take a walk — all of which are examples of ways we are meeting *physical* needs. Although temporarily it may give us a sense of relief — because of the benefits it gives to the body, — if we are really paying attention, we know that these approaches did not resolve the underlying psychological tension. Likewise, if we are venting our unresolved frustration and anger through vigorous exercise, we may end up being fit and looking really good, but our resentment will seep through other areas of our lives in passive-aggressive ways (which are the ways of *silent resentment*).

So even though we may be doing *something* to address the anger, the outcome of that will not be effective, for the very simple reason that it wouldn't be the *right* solution. And what happens when we don't have the right solution?

Our needs persist.

And it shows.

It shows in how we feel.

When psychological needs persist, our emotional signals will grow in their intensity. When we deny what we feel (or do things to make the feeling go away) and do not have a chance to explore what we truly need, the discomfort continues to build up internally resulting in emotional tension. And that is a sure clue that we did not get the right outcome from the way we went about it.

The world is a noisy place. The world of the material especially so. And so it is easy to get distracted and misdirected with everything that is coming at you and is offered to you. Many of these offers (e.g., stuff you see in ads, various products and services marketed to you) distract you from your real needs by meeting your *wants* instead. The constant meeting of the wants is an endless cycle of wanting even more. You see, despite all the consumption, the satisfaction of wants is superficial, shallow, and not long-lasting, because it does not actually respond to what is truly needed.

So what do we truly need?

How do we get the outcomes we seek?

First of all, be OK with it being a trial and error process, especially in the beginning stages of getting to know yourself. The longer you have been running away from your feelings, the more time will be needed to truly get to know yourself and your needs. But guess what? In seeing what doesn't work for us, we still gain valuable knowledge about ourselves, because knowing ourselves includes both — knowing what works and what doesn't. Outcomes we do not like will truly help us hone in even more precisely on what *does* work for us.

Whereas identifying a need comes down to one of the 8 Core Psychological Needs, meeting the identified need is about knowing yourself and what works for you. Let's take a physical need as an example. You may identify that you are feeling tired and you need rest. Great! But what kind of rest you need depends on your unique situation.

Meaning, do you need a break from work and switch to something else? Or is this about wrapping things up and calling it a day? Are you tired in a way that requires a good night's sleep? Or, are you tired because you've been sitting too long and need to move? You see, what kind of "tired" you are will depend on the unique expression and manifestation of your need, in your particular situation, and at that moment in time. So tuning into yourself and asking yourself questions (e.g., "What is making me tired?" or "What do I need in order to feel rested?" and so on) will guide *you* towards finding a proper resource and a way of meeting this need that is appropriate for *you*. Although this is an example of finding the right answer for a physical need, we follow the same process for psychological needs. This also means that:

Only you can tell if your need is met.

Only you know if the outcome is right for you.

Because only you know — how you feel.

Knowing how you feel requires not only self-awareness, but also a certain degree of honesty with ourselves. We have to be honest with ourselves as to whether the way we go about our needs is actually meeting them. We have to be honest about our emotions as well. Did we or did we not restore equilibrium and bring ourselves back to balance? Are we wasting our resources on the wants and superficial desires at the expense of our needs?

Only you would know what outcomes you are getting. And your trusted and reliable clue to this is — your emotions and how you feel. If your emotions feel resolved and that sense of balance is sustained, then it is likely that you have met the need. If not, you have to re-evaluate your approach and try something else. You may find the following questions helpful as you assess the outcome:

- Is my need met?
- Does the situation feel resolved?

- Am I clear about my needs?
- Is there anything else I need to do about it?
- How have I met this need before?
- Has it been successful?
- What else can I try?
- What other choices do I have?
- How else can I take care of myself?
- What other needs may be involved?

It may also be helpful to work your way through the 3-Step Needs-Based Process once again to fully comprehend your situation. It may give you a better sense of awareness around what the trigger was, what you were feeling, and what needs were implicated. By revisiting the three steps of the Needs-Based Process, you may gain new insights, which will help you either better understand your needs or the options and resources available to you.

One thing to watch out for when evaluating outcomes and monitoring our emotional resonance with the actions we take is this: judging the process as opposed to looking at the outcome. What I mean by that is that we have to be mindful not to confuse how we feel about the process of getting to the outcome (which may not be pleasant) with the outcome itself (a satisfied need).

For example, you may not be enjoying broccoli, and so the process of eating it may not be giving you wonderful sensations. However, if it has satiated you and resolved your hunger, then the outcome of that process is positive. Meaning, you have met your need. Likewise, you may not be feeling like doing it every time you exercise, but you know your body needs it, and so you are doing it. In other words, we are not trying to satisfy the process — although we may certainly enjoy it whenever possible — but the need. Putting in extra effort in making the process fun and *forcing* yourself to enjoy it when you really don't is not going to make you enjoy it any more, and that is OK.

There is no need to lie to ourselves. Some processes may not be enjoyable, and it is what it is. If that's the case, simply focus on the outcomes *at the end* of the process. Once the process is complete, that is a good time to assess whether the outcome was functional, which is to say — whether the need was met. Although the process of meeting our needs may not always be fun, having needs met will always feel good.

It is important, therefore, to judge the outcome based on whether the need is met, as opposed to whether getting there was fun and easy. You can always improve the process of getting there once you find better ways to go about it, which also means — finding better resources.

Another very common example I see is this one: When it comes to housework or chores so many people are being told that these things can and should be fun (and that it's up to us to make them so) and if they're not fun, then we're doing them wrong. So now on top of an unpleasant task, you also feel bad about yourself. Why do that? Stop trying to make mundane things fun. It's too much work to do the chore *and* to also make sure you are having fun doing it. It's OK. You can meet your need for fun elsewhere, with things that are truly fun for you. And those other things, like chores, do not have to be enjoyable.

In other words, we should stop trying hard to make them so. Why? Because that's a waste of energy. Some of them cannot be fun, no matter how much you try (like cleaning puke after your sick children), so don't waste your energy there.

Let's just accept this simple truth: one task cannot carry the burden of fulfilling every single one of our needs. Some things will fulfill the need for fun and enjoyment. Others will bring meaning and purpose. And still others — like chores — will simply fulfill the need for order, safety, hygiene, and so on. Most of the mundane tasks and chores are the ones that have to do with basic maintenance and our physical needs. A lot of them may feel really boring and tedious, because let's be honest — we are more than our bodies and our physical needs. So instead of thinking "how can I make this fun" focus on simply getting them done. Tell yourself that you understand your needs and you, as a responsible adult, decided to attend to your needs even when the process of getting there may not be as fulfilling. The outcome of meeting the need always is.

Even when the process is not fun, it is the outcome that we are after.

While you focus on getting the outcome you need, it also helps if you remember to acknowledge and validate how you feel about the task or the process of getting there, because that does always make us feel better. It helps us be seen and heard — which is another one of our core needs — even if it's just us talking to ourselves in our own head.

Of course, when it comes to unpleasant tasks, no one is stopping us from asking — how can we make it easier? How can we make it less unpleasant? On the practical side of things, if dreadful tasks take up too much of your energy, do think about what can be done about them to change them. Or think about what else needs to come into your life to create a bit more balance between things you like and don't like doing. Understandably, this book cannot offer solutions for everything because everyone's needs and resources would be different. However, if you do wish that the process of doing something was easier, here are a few questions to start with:

- What is another way of doing this?
- Is there a better time/place to do this?
- Is this the only way to get this need met?
- What would I be willing to do instead of this?

It's also worth noting that, as our needs change, the need for certain tasks or chores will also change. Some of the tasks will go away and new ones may become a necessity. Because of that, every once in a while, it helps to revisit our habits to make sure we are not doing things on autopilot, especially those that are no longer needed.

In any case, lying to ourselves and pretending we enjoy the things we don't like takes up a lot of mental energy and, therefore, it depletes our resources. It is completely unnecessary. We can validate the fact that certain things are boring and yet that we do them to take care of ourselves. Even though we may not appreciate the process, we do appreciate the outcome. So any time you find the process to be boring, annoying, etc., shift your attention to the outcome and the *why* behind it. And that reason is — to meet a particular need.

This way you will see the value of the process. It brings you closer to the outcomes you want.

Chapter 7

Unmet Needs, Neglect, & Need-to-Care

So far in this book we talked about how essential your needs are and how important it is to make sure they are met. In this chapter, I'd like to offer a few thoughts on what happens when our needs are *not* met. There is something we talked about earlier that will be important to keep in mind here, given the focus of this chapter. And that is, the difference between needs and wants. Knowing this difference makes the process of meeting our needs easier, since there are way fewer needs than there are wants. There are also many more ways in which we are able to meet the needs, as opposed to the wants, because what we want is sometimes so very specific that it limits our ability to satisfy it right away.

Knowing that our essential needs can be met in many different ways is very helpful because it gives us options and can help us see alternatives and compromises, which is especially important when our resources may be limited. When we can distinguish wants from needs we can breathe easier, knowing that it is not necessary to focus on fulfilling every wish and desire, especially if we do that at the expense of our needs.

As long as we are focusing on our needs, we are doing a good job of taking care of ourselves. And that leads to a sustainable sense of wellbeing and vitality.

Although we already talked about the distinction between wants and needs, it may be helpful to illustrate it one more time with an example. Let's start with an example of a physical need and let's say you are noticing that you're hungry, which signals that you have a need for food. There are many ways in which you can meet that need. If you are thinking something like "I want mashed potatoes and green beans" that is an expression of a *want*, a particular *preference,* which requires very specific resources (i.e., mashed potatoes and green beans). If you have them around — great! You can satisfy both your need and your want. But if you don't, that's also OK, because there are other things you could eat. If you eat something other than mashed potatoes and green beans, you have satisfied your need, which also means you took care of yourself.

Where we make the mistake is we forgo *the need* in favor of pursuing *a want* and do not realize that this is what we are doing. Staying with the food example, what this will look like is deciding to eat nothing else, unless it is specifically what we want, and go on without eating until mashed potatoes and green beans become available. Although something like this is less likely to happen with our physical needs (since, as we previously discussed, we are better at meeting them), it is, nonetheless, something that happens quite often with our psychological needs. We may put too much emphasis on our preferences, while failing to meet our basic needs.

What also tends to be the case with our psychological needs is that we are meeting the wrong needs all the time. Why is this happening? Because we lack proper understanding of our needs (see Chapter 5 for conversation about Need Awareness) and are not very skilled at meeting them (see Chapter 6 for conversation about Resources Awareness). Since we have discussed all of these points in more detail in the previous chapters, I will not reiterate them here. However, the reason why I am mentioning them is because of the end results we are getting.

And that is — neglected needs.

But you may be wondering, "So what? How serious is it really?" What happens when our needs are *not* met? And if it really is so bad that it requires its own chapter, then is there a way to correct the course? So yes, it is serious. And yes, there are things we can do to get back on track.

Neglecting your needs comes at a cost to your wellbeing.

It's a big deal.

And that is why we need to talk about it.

THREE REASONS BEHIND UNMET NEEDS

To prevent the problem of unmet needs to begin with, we have to understand *why* we neglect our needs. There is always a reason. Broadly speaking, there are three reasons why we may end up with unmet needs.

The first one is our beliefs around needs and whether we think negatively about them. The second reason is lack of awareness. Meaning, even though we may have a favorable perspective about needs, we may still lack a good understanding of them. When we do not understand our needs and are not aware of them, we are more likely to neglect them or, at best, meet them incidentally rather than intentionally. And the final reason for unmet needs is because we don't know *how* to meet them or don't access appropriate resources for us. Let's take a closer look at each of these reasons:

1. Beliefs about needs

Here is how our beliefs about needs get in the way of meeting them. If we believe that needs make us "needy" or that it is a sign of weakness, we will deny that we have needs and try to overcome them with various mantras and affirmations (e.g., "I am not a burden to myself and others"). We may believe that, as social creatures, our main purpose is to serve others and, therefore, we put other people's needs ahead of our own (e.g., "I am not a taker, I am a giver"). Because of these beliefs we end up ignoring our own needs and, consequently, fail to meet them.

For those of us who do this, the danger is that we get good at dulling the pain of unmet needs and at denying that it's there. In other words, when unmet needs generate discomfort, distress, and even despair — which they inevitably do as this is your systems' way of signaling S.O.S. to you (i.e., "please pay attention!") — we may interpret those signals as requiring us to be even "tougher." So not only do we deny our needs, we also deny the pain those unmet needs cause. But this can only last so long before it eventually leads to dire consequences, like mental health issues and/or addiction problems.

By developing greater awareness, not only we can get ahead of these consequences and prevent them, but also — and more importantly — we get to live more fulfilling and happy lives, because we are actually attending to ourselves and getting what we need. Meeting our needs means giving ourselves life energy. It is *the only way* we can sustain ourselves.

From this perspective, fulfilling your needs is not a frivolous or privileged act. This is one of the things that is so wrong with our culture these days, where almost every conversation — even when it has to do with meeting our basic needs — turns into a conversation about privilege. No, meeting your needs is not a privilege, it is a right. A basic human right.

If you carry these beliefs about needs, you've got it backwards. When we think that the only people who can meet their needs are the ones that have access to certain privileges, we are disempowering ourselves by adopting a perspective that ultimately does not serve us. Although life is not easy and we have to be intentional and proactive about seeking appropriate resources, it is our responsibility to do so. When we believe that only "privileged" people can do that, we place that responsibility in someone else's hands. Sure, well-to-do individuals may have more resources or more choices when it comes to meeting their needs, and yet those who live within different means can *also* meet their needs. They just do it differently. We have to shift our perspective to be able to see that.

When we talk ourselves out of our responsibility to meet our needs (because of our beliefs), we are inevitably engaging in self-neglect. Neglect of the needs is neglect of the Self as *a whole being* (not just the body). When we don't acknowledge the whole spectrum of our needs, we get disconnected from ourselves. If we only attend to the needs of the body, we lose the sense of who we are. Loss of the sense of Self leads to loss of meaning, which then leads to a personal crisis.

In order to know our needs, we have to ask questions about them. But to ask questions about them, we first have to acknowledge that our needs matter.

2. Lack of awareness

But let's say you don't have disempowering beliefs about your needs. Is that enough to meet them? Not quite. Even though we may believe needs are natural and valid, or that our needs do matter and require attending to, we may still lack awareness of what our needs are.

We may not sense it when needs arise.

We may not have good knowledge of ourselves. It may be that our lives are too noisy or too fast and we don't slow down enough to listen and tune into what we need. It may also be the case that we misinterpret emotions and, instead of seeing them as signals for needs, we perceive them as errors in our thinking (something we discussed in Chapter 2).

When we lack awareness, then even if we do sense a need, we may not have the clarity as to what it is speaking to within us. Is it a need for *attention* or for *meaning*? Are we seeking to *connect* or to have an *impact*? Do we need more *fun* and *enjoyment* in our lives or a clearer sense of *purpose*? Which one is it? When we are not aware of ourselves enough or do not understand our specific needs, we are more likely to neglect them or, at best, meet them incidentally, by chance.

If what I'm saying here resonates with you and you have a hunch that this may be the reason your needs are not met, then there are several things you can do. To resolve these challenges we have to first realize that we have not been paying enough attention to ourselves, and then follow the three steps of the Needs-Based Process. The only way to feel good and balanced is through meeting our needs, both proactively on a regular basis, as well as when emotions let us know of a need arising in the present moment.

You can also become more intentional about getting to know yourself and your needs. This means asking more questions about your *emotions*, because emotions signal to us about our needs and that is the perfect place to start. Questions like "What am I feeling?" "What is making me feel this way?" "What is the trigger?" and "What do I need?" — are all good starting points. Revisit Chapter 4 "Step One: Emotion Awareness" for a more detailed explanation.

In addition to that, it helps to spend quiet time reflecting and checking in with yourself across all 8 Core Psychological Needs (see Appendix B for a list of basic needs). This may look like asking questions such as: "Out of these eight domains, which ones feel fulfilled and which ones seem lacking?" or "How am I meeting my need for *Growth*? Is there something I need in this area?" or "What is filling me up when it comes to *Connection*? Am I doing enough of that?" and so on.

- Needs exist whether or not we are paying attention to them.
- It only serves us to pay more attention.
- When we pay attention, we are more likely to meet our needs.

You can begin by paying attention to what is already within your area of awareness. Build from there. What else is calling your attention? How might you want to respond to that? What will serve you and your needs? That is how we begin to know ourselves better and increase our self-awareness.

3. Lack of appropriate resources

And the final most common reason for unmet needs is lack of resources to meet them. This may be happening when we don't know *how* to meet a particular need or can't seem to find resources to do so, which ultimately means — it gets neglected. So even if we don't struggle with unhelpful beliefs and even when we are keenly aware of our needs, we may still run into a situation where we either do not have access to resources or have a need/resource mismatch for whatever reason. It may also be the case that, perhaps, something that might have worked for us in the past doesn't work for us anymore. Or something we used to have access to previously is no longer available.

This may be happening due to changes in the external environment or due to personal and internal adjustments. If we take a need for *Meaning*, for example, it may be that it is not currently met because you were just laid off from a job you really loved and found a lot of meaning in. This is an example of external changes. Or perhaps, it is because the job you used to love is no longer meaningful due to personal shifts and changes in your internal world (e.g., redefining your values).

So even if we have a solid understanding of ourselves, are good at paying attention to what we need, and are generally consistent at doing things proactively, even then, sometimes there will be situations outside of our control where our needs exceed resources available to us at that moment. And so, in the above example, since the need for meaning can no longer be fulfilled through that job, we must look for something else that can serve as the new source of meaning for us. The answer as to what that new source will be is different for every person, because it depends on what we find meaningful (and what, in particular, used to be so meaningful and fulfilling about that job).

And so you may have unmet needs, but it isn't for the lack of trying, that's for sure. What do you do then? First of all, you must acknowledge the facts. Acknowledge the situation itself and how it is impacting your needs. This allows the need to stay top-of-mind. We also must acknowledge that even though there may not be available resources at the moment, our needs are still important and valid, and that we will do our best to fulfill the need as soon as the opportunity to do so presents itself. By validating our needs, we affirm and validate *ourselves*.

Without that, we risk slipping into need denial, whereby we tell ourselves that the need is no longer important because resources to meet it are not available. Need denial, whatever its cause, has serious consequences, as I already mentioned. We have to validate ourselves and our needs, and acknowledge the level of discomfort — and perhaps even suffering — that we may be experiencing while our needs are not being met. The level of discomfort may depend on whether the situation is relatively new and temporary, whether it has been prolonged and is ongoing, and whether the need is pressing or not. Regardless of the magnitude of the need, though, we have to accept it, because there is no such thing as a need that's not valid.

Although the reality of our life may be such that a particular need may not be prioritized (due to other more pressing needs) or be delayed due to lack of resources, this does not diminish its significance. Acknowledgement of our situation and validation of our needs, despite the situation we're in, allows us to put in continuous effort towards finding new resources. In addition to that, this acknowledgement and validation protects us against dysfunctional outcomes.

However, if we stay here too long, without resources to meet our needs, it does eventually lead to burnout, loss of vitality, loss of life force, energy, etc. Just like with our physical needs, in that we can't live on air and sunshine alone, the same applies to psychological needs. We cannot ignore or forget them, or promise ourselves indefinitely that "someday" we will attend to what really matters. Now that you know the reasons for unmet needs, let's take a look at what happens to an unmet need over time.

THE UNMET NEEDS ARC

As I mentioned earlier, the problem with needs is not that we have them, but that we disregard them. In other words, your needs are not your problems, your problems are your *unmet needs*. What this means is that all unmet needs result in poor personal outcomes and compromise our wellbeing.

It may be helpful to know that the negative consequences of unmet needs do not happen immediately. There is a certain trajectory of events that unfold over time that, not only helps you understand what happens with an unmet need as the time goes on, but also allows you to be more mindful and intervene as soon as you can.

Regardless of whether the needs are ignored intentionally (due to beliefs and attitudes about them) or unintentionally (due to lack of awareness or resources), when they are unmet, they will follow a curved trajectory that is shaped like an arc. Let me remind you that core basic needs (as opposed to wishes and wants) — do persist and intensify over time if they are left unattended to. Unlike wishes and wants that are more-or-less fleeting, needs do not go away and will keep sending signals, until they are met. So when the needs are not met, they will generate tension that will continue to create discomfort within our bodies and minds. This escalation of intensity has a functional purpose of generating more awareness and more energy to propel us towards taking care of them.

Thirst or hunger, for example, will preoccupy us, causing physical and even cognitive symptoms, making it impossible to concentrate on what we are doing. This is so that we drop what we are doing and attend to our needs for food or water. A child who is really hungry may show additional symptoms in a form of emotional dysregulation, like a tantrum. Even adults note a similar tendency to become, as they say, "*hangry*" (angry because of hunger). All of these are examples of a need intensifying as it moves through an arc trajectory. If this situation is prolonged, this unmet need will lead to exhaustion, fatigue, and eventually to passing out (when left unattended for too long in extreme cases).

This arc trajectory of escalation applies to the needs across the whole spectrum, not only to physical needs. A person whose *psychological* needs are neglected, will also show *somatic* symptoms in addition to signs of emotional distress. Adults who are chronically "stressed" — a sure sign of prolonged state of unmet needs — experience both psychological and physical tension in their bodies (e.g., pain in the neck, back, or shoulders, digestive issues, etc.). So whether we are talking about physical or psychological needs, they are interconnected in how the built-up tension shows up.

The purpose behind this tension is to make us pay attention, to make us stop what we are doing. It urges us to attend to the needs we have. This function is there because, unlike the wants, needs are actually vital to our physical and psychological survival. In other words, we will not pass out if we don't get a *particular flavor* of vitamin water (i.e., unfulfilled *want*), but we will pass out without *any* water (i.e., unfulfilled *need*).

When a need is present, the tension rises to make an organism take action to meet the need. If the need is not met and is ignored, it eventually leads to all systems going S.O.S. and after that — if the need is still not met — to an eventual shutdown. This is because sustained and persistent tension can be taxing on the body as a whole, if left unresolved for too long, and so it will eventually drop off and lead to withdrawal. Physically that may look like passing out and psychologically it may look like detachment, disconnect, and suppression. This inevitably leads to burnout, loss of vitality, and loss of sense of aliveness. We will talk more about that later in this chapter.

The withdrawal happens due to the neurological signaling in the brain that there aren't enough resources in the environment and that, for whatever reason, we are not able to replenish energy reserves in our physical and psychological systems. And so, in order to preserve the organism as a whole, the brain will "crisis-manage" the situation by down-regulating certain functions in order to conserve energy. This stops the process of seeking resources for the time being, since it hasn't been effective at that moment, until another opportunity presents itself in the future. To better understand this, a good analogy here is like when you call a customer service line and you are being put on hold. If you are waiting for too long to have your call answered, you are eventually going to "withdraw your request" by hanging up. The call may have ended, but it doesn't mean that your needs were addressed. It means that you waited too long and it wasn't worth exerting any more effort at that point, and you will try again later.

The difference between this example and how the brain manages a situation of an unmet need is the degree of awareness and intentionality on our part. In other words, whereas in the customer service call analogy it is we who intentionally decide to "withdraw the request," when it comes to our physical and psychological needs — it is the brain.

Since we are the ones who are failing to meet the needs, the management of energy demands unconsciously gets passed onto our nervous system and automatic processes in the brain. At that point it becomes more of a process that happens outside of our awareness. However, the more aware we are of the pressing need and the more intentional we are of trying to meet it, the less likely it is that the withdrawal will happen. Just like, you are more likely to stay on the line, if someone from the customer service center is periodically checking in with you while you wait to get your concerns addressed.

I created a diagram to help you visualize what the arc looks like. It is important to understand that the arc of the unmet need (the bold line with arrows) represents the intensity of its signaling and our degree of awareness about it.

The higher the need travels up the curve in its escalation, the more aware we are of the need itself and the more urgency there is behind satisfying it. After a certain period of time, however, if the need is not met, the signal begins to travel down the curve as an expression of our diminishing awareness about it.

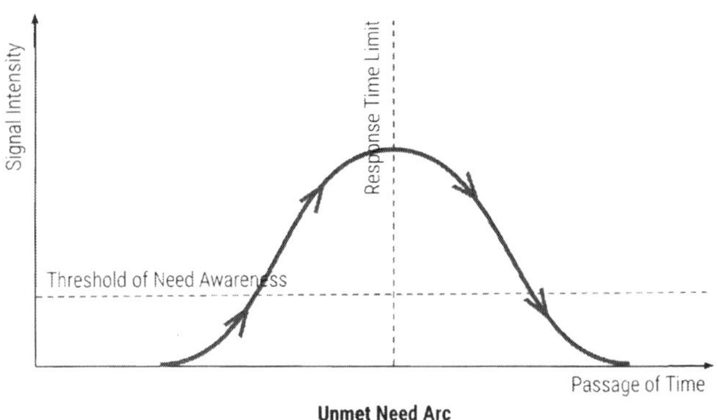

Unmet Need Arc

This is not to be confused with the relevance and importance of the need itself. What I mean is, the arc represents our awareness of the need and the intensity with which it is felt. As the need travels past the limit of reasonable response time (i.e., our failure to address it in a timely manner), the downcurve does not represent a diminishing need, but is rather an expression of our *diminishing awareness* about it. As our awareness wanes, the need moves into the background of our existence, creating a low but persistent sense of discontent and discomfort.

The less aware we are and the less active we are in meeting our needs' demands, the more likely it is that those unanswered requests will be withdrawn beyond our threshold of awareness. As a result, in self-preservation mode, the brain will direct certain functions of our psyche or our body (depending on the nature of the need) to shut down or be put in a state of hibernation, if you will. Sounds pretty severe, these are scary things, right?

This is what happens in extreme cases and occurs as a result of a gradual build-up of tension surrounding neglected needs. Our organism does that as an adaptive response to conditions of resource scarcity with the goal of preserving whatever energy it has left.

Since you are reading this book, I am assuming you care enough about yourself to never get to that state of neglect. However, I am mentioning this here so that you can get a sense of the whole arc and know where you are along that trajectory when addressing your needs. This is why, as I have explained earlier, when we have preferences (i.e., wants and wishes), they normally will fade into the background and below our threshold of awareness, so that the underlying need can become more clear and turn into the ultimate driver of exploring options. In the environment of low resources, our mind's focus will shift from a specific want to a core need, which — in contrast to a specific preference — will be easier to meet by whatever means are available.

And that is the arc of unmet needs.

We go from a baseline of a balanced functioning to a bit of discomfort, to a gradual increase in tension, to distress. If the need is not attended to at this point, it may escalate to despair, before it eventually passes through the threshold of response time and declines into a "giving up" mode. In the worst case scenario, when we neglect our psychological needs, it leads to a quiet kind of "quitting on oneself," disconnecting from ourselves, our sense of aliveness, and what we are all about.

When the level of distress is the strongest, it is usually the clearest and the loudest signal about what is missing and what is needed. It is also the moment that requires the most direct and intentional action from us, because the time window to respond to that need is closing before our awareness of it begins to decline (due to lack of response).

In contrast to that, the stage of quiet quitting is where we feel "blah" or constantly irritated but don't know why. This lack of knowing is precisely the outcome of diminished awareness. This is the stage where our needs have become nearly invisible to us, and our sense of Self — barely tangible. The "Why am I angry all the time?" question is a sign of that muffled pain of unmet needs pushed out of the way and into the background of our noisy existence.

Let's also note that there absolutely will be times when we cannot meet our needs for whatever reason.

That is unavoidable.

However, we must never lose sight of them.

No matter how good we are at responding to our needs overall, there will be times when we are not able to. Maybe we are dealing with a lot, maybe we got carried away and forgot to pay attention, maybe we are unwell, or have to take care of others. Whatever the case may be. Hopefully these situations are far and few in between and that, when they do happen, we are taking note of why, in order to make sure we do what is in our control and make any changes necessary to manage similar situations better going forward.

Still, since times like that will happen, there is no reason to panic. It is OK. It is what we choose *to do with these situations* that truly matters and makes a big difference. Let's look at a couple of simple examples of unmet needs.

These may be minor situations, like when you realize how boring your whole day has been running soul-sucking errands and that you would like to do something fun. You may not be able to entertain yourself at that moment, so what do you do? Instead of pulling out your phone as a means of distraction, which will not truly meet your underlying need, you may think of a plan to do something you truly find enjoyable, once you get home.

Or, let's say you are driving and feeling really hungry but it will take some time to get to your destination. Instead of grabbing a bag of chips, you are willing to wait a little longer to get home where you can get yourself a proper nutritious meal. So even though your need cannot be met right away, you are acknowledging it as important and valid, and are planning how to attend to it. This way you are staying aware of your needs and are making intentional plans about them.

These are examples of what I call "minor incidents" when isolated needs occur in-the-moment and cannot be met there and then. It is not necessary to satisfy our needs immediately, as we are resilient enough to wait, within reason, to get our needs met. But there also may be more complex situations where many needs may be implicated and are not being met over an extended period of time. And so, given the range of situations where needs may not be met, we can think of them as landing on a continuum of less frequent and less intense to more frequent and more intense incidents.

An example of a prolonged intense scenario, where needs go on unmet, could be a situation that your whole family is facing, like a serious illness, loss of financial stability, natural disaster, etc. Going through a very stressful time may diminish a number of our resources all at once (financial, social, emotional, time, etc.).

The need for safety, which is usually met through stability, predictability, and routine may be compromised when we are going through a series of chaotic transitions. We can expect that several needs may go unmet in times of crises. Some situations of significant loss and trauma can destabilize our mental wellbeing and our sense of Self, due to prolonged lack of care for the needs and for the Self.

Although these situations are rare, it is important to know that there are consequences to prolonged experiences of unmet needs, and will require some recovery time. Recovery takes place when we begin to take care of our needs again, slowly but surely pulling ourselves out of a depleted state and out of misery. How long this takes depends on how long we have experienced deprivation and neglect of needs. It is important to know that this isn't anything we won't be able to correct with proper attention, dedicated care, and at times — professional support. However, patience is also required, because recovery from neglected needs does not work like a switch, automatically and without effort.

But let's take a deep breath...

Although I am giving you a heads up about what might happen in the worst case scenario, things aren't usually that bad on a day-to-day basis. Our internal world and sense of worth will not collapse if, per our earlier examples, we can't feed ourselves right away or do something fun as soon as we feel bored.

Usually we have some degree of resilience and are able to tolerate a certain level of discomfort, and we are able to wait to meet our needs properly instead of doing something impulsive in the moment (like eating chips or scrolling on social media). But besides planning to do something in the future about the needs that cannot be met on the spot (which is true for most of them), there is one more thing that makes all the difference as to whether unmet needs escalate and whether they will follow the arc all the way down into the zone of withdrawal.

And that leads us to the next segment of this chapter, the "need-to-care" concept.

NEED-TO-CARE

This is something we've briefly talked about before, but it is so essential — especially when there is a significant delay in meeting our needs — that it requires a little bit more attention. I am talking about the acknowledgement and the validation of our needs. Acknowledging our needs to ourselves is the only way to stay in-sight of our needs and to stay *visible to ourselves*. Without that, our needs will go into hiding and will play out in subconscious ways by seeking resources inappropriately, at the expense of ourselves and others. And that leads to dysfunction, self-sabotage, and a build up of defense mechanisms.

Failure not only to meet our needs but also to *acknowledge* to ourselves that this is the reality of our current situation declares our needs as unimportant. And this will prevent us from searching for resources in a proper way, because this lack of acknowledgement pushes needs out of our conscious awareness. Since they are no longer in-focus, we drop intentional efforts to get what we need. On the other hand, validation of our needs brings them back into our awareness, makes us care, and makes sure we attend to them. As living breathing organisms, we have needs that have to be cared for. In other words, we have a need for care, and that is what the need-to-care concept is about.

When needs are not met, at the very least — we have to validate them. That is to say, we *need to care* that we have them. This is the bare minimum we can and should do. We have to explicitly acknowledge what is going on instead of dismissing the needs, simply because we were not able to meet them. This protects us from thinking that our needs are not important and, therefore, that we are also not important and not worthy of our own care, attention, resources, etc. In other words, it protects us from *dismissing ourselves*. Through validation we tell ourselves: "I see you, I see your needs, hang in there. Your needs are valid and important and you, too, are worthy and important. As soon as I am able, I will take care of these needs."

This isn't a silly little thing to do *only if* you have time for it.

No. This is an absolute must when we have unmet needs.

Another thing to understand is that this acknowledgement cannot be done in a superficial way. If it is, it will come off as ingenuine and will have the same effect as dismissing yourself. The last thing we need is to engage in self-mockery. We know when we don't mean what we say and there is no point in lying to ourselves. That is the opposite of what is required here. We have to leverage the powerful tool of validation, especially when we do not have the ability to meet our needs, since that may be all that we are able to offer ourselves for the time being.

Seeing ourselves is non-negotiable.

And we have to do a good job with it.

So slow down and let yourself know that you do care about yourself and about your needs. You see them. You see yourself in need of something and you will do your best to get yourself what you need as soon as possible. This is important because, no matter how much we may deny it, deep down — beyond all other needs — we do have a *need to care* about ourselves.

Meeting our needs is the way we nurture ourselves. So when we don't have resources in that particular moment to meet our needs, validating is the next best thing we can do to nurture ourselves. Even when we do not have resources to meet whatever need it may be, by way of validating ourselves and our needs, we are actually meeting another important need of ours — that of self-acceptance, self-acknowledgement, and self-worth.

Acceptance of ourselves, our needs, wants, thoughts, emotions, the full range of our experience, as well as anything and everything that comes with the very experience of not having our needs met in that moment... All of that is how we are being seen. Being seen is vital to our wellbeing, especially when other needs are not being met. It preserves the integrity of our Self, which is built on the sense of importance and worth.

In spending time on validation and acknowledgement, it helps us preserve our own integrity and our own personal relationship with ourselves. Because, instead of dismissing who we are and our needs as unimportant, we are staying connected with ourselves and reassuring ourselves of our commitment to our whole being and to our responsibility to take care of ourselves. In other words, when all else fails, when nothing else can be done, the one thing that holds us together is *the need-to-care* — the need to care for ourselves, to stay visible to ourselves.

Needless to say, this need-to-care approach has to be used in a sincere manner. We cannot use acknowledgement and validation as an escape from our responsibilities or as a way of avoiding ourselves and our needs.

If we are constantly unable to show up for ourselves and meet our core needs (both physical and psychological), then we have to pause and explore why. What may be going on? When we tell ourselves that we are worthy and important and those words are not backed up by action of meeting our needs on a regular basis, eventually these words will do more harm than good and break our own self-trust.

No matter all the promises we make to ourselves to take care of ourselves and our needs, if we fail to actually make it happen, we eventually burn out. In the end, it will deeply invalidate us. So in order for the need-to-care approach to work, the acknowledgement and validation have to come from a genuine place and be followed by action as soon as possible. Otherwise, you will have an experience that is similar to a situation when you are indefinitely put on-hold on a customer service line. Even though a robotic voice tells you every two minutes that you are a "valuable customer" and someone will be with you in "just a moment," after half an hour of that, you will detest hearing any such recognition and see it as meaningless and frustrating.

BEWARE OF BURNOUT

As human beings, we are quite resilient. We don't just fall apart and break down if our needs are not met immediately. Perhaps, you've seen children do that, and that is because they do not have enough experience and perspective to know that their needs will be met, and that they just have to wait a little bit. As we get older and become adults, we acquire a lot of that experience, which supports our capacity to keep going in the face of adversity. We can also tap into other capacities to hold on to (such as need-to-care, for example) until we have the opportunity to satisfy our needs. However, regardless of how much perseverance and resilience one has, it does have a limit, and there is only so much we can endure without actually taking care of ourselves.

When our needs are not met for long stretches of time, we inevitably burn out. And no wonder why. If you really think about it, you will see that what happens when we attend to our needs is that we get energy to move on and move ahead. Satisfying our needs results in vitality and strengthens our sense of aliveness, whereas with neglected needs — we have no life force and get depleted.

Burnout is the outcome of prolonged neglect, self-neglect in particular. We arrive here at the final stages of the unmet needs arc. Burnout happens because of an assumption, perhaps, that we can last longer without attending to ourselves than is actually possible. One look at our energy levels, our sense of wellbeing and vitality, tells us everything we need to know. It is hard to feel satiated from a place of depletion. If you have been neglecting yourself for a while, it will take time to get back to optimal functioning and learn to trust yourself again. It will take time to rebuild that connection with yourself and to get to know who you are, what matters to you, what your needs are, and how they can be met.

If you don't like the idea of feeling bad all the time, you've got to understand that the way out is through taking care of your needs. If you don't, you will feel the way you don't want to feel.

Those who take care of others are even more likely to burn out.

If you are a caretaker, pay close attention. When other less-able people depend on us, it is natural to want to put them first, and we often do. If we are not careful, we run out of steam meeting their needs before we ever get to ourselves. So if you have little children or aging parents, a partner who is seriously ill, and so on, this part of our conversation is especially important for you. Taking care of others is demanding enough even when we show up rested and taken care of. Imagine what happens when we do all that with our own cup always empty.

Not having our own needs met means that the impact from other people's needs and demands will be even higher than normal. And because of that, we get depleted exponentially faster.

In other words, you are not just burning the candle, but you're burning it from both ends, as they say. Things that might have taken less energy, now demand even more. The less energy we have to give, the more energy it will take from us to do anything — that is the irony of burnout. This happens because the gap between what is required and what you've got keeps growing bigger and bigger, becoming more and more taxing on all of your systems.

As caring empathetic people, it is second nature for us to slip into an auto-pilot mode, where we get pulled by everyone else's needs. Not only do we end up putting ourselves second, we rarely find intentional time to do what our heart is asking us to do. Once in a while, as an exception, this approach of "others first, me last" can work, but when it becomes a way of living, it leads to burnout.

- As they say, we cannot give to others what we do not have.

How can we have energy for others, if we don't have it within us? How can we be peaceful, compassionate, and attentive to others, when we are not that way with ourselves?

Most of us have heard about or have experienced some form of burnout. Oftentimes it comes up in conversations about work when, let's say, a job becomes too demanding, tasks are piling up, and to-do lists keep growing. We may feel totally exhausted both mentally and physically after what used to be a normal day at work. But let's be clear, when we are talking about burnout that comes as a result of unmet needs, this isn't the kind of exhaustion that goes away after a good night's rest. It is the kind of exhaustion that feels like complete and total loss of life energy, a sense of deadness inside, a loss of our sense of aliveness. Nothing feels doable and there is no sense of what can help. Sounds like depression, and it can certainly turn into one if things continue to roll in the same direction.

Burnout is a manifestation of a *depressive state of being* and it is a result of a systemic problem of low energy, vitality, and motivation. And when I say systemic, I don't mean in terms of our society and how it functions, but rather the way we run our own lives and the way we respond to our internal systems of functioning (i.e., the way we respond to internal signals, our awareness of emotions, of our needs, etc.).

While we can find a way to walk away from demanding people, places, and things, we cannot walk away from our needs. Nor can we walk away from how we treat ourselves.

When our needs are not met, our energy is low. If it is not replenished, we burn out to a full stop. That level of self-neglect is quite dangerous and will require a long recovery time, as we have discussed in the previous section, the Unmet Needs Arc. It is the satisfaction and the fulfillment of our own needs that gives us energy and the capacity to face life demands, which may or may not include taking care of others.

The way you can tell what kind of exhaustion you are feeling and whether it is coming from burnout is — once again — by checking in with your emotions. Our lives are busy, and there are many physically exhausting days. Just the amount of physical movement and the actual tasks that get done throughout the day can leave us completely spent and ready for bed. But it is important to note the emotional tone of that exhaustion. As our head hits the pillows, are we still pretty satisfied with our day, or are we irritated about everything in our lives and feel resentful that all we did that day was run around helping other people? If the exhaustion is physical, a good night's rest will help, but if it is burnout from unmet needs, then sleep alone will not restore us back to capacity.

Burnout does not go away on its own.

It requires intentional effort.

There is no pill or bandaid for this problem. Without intentional effort, it only gets more and more severe. Being intentional about recovering from and preventing burnout means becoming fully committed to taking care of our needs, both physical and psychological. Unless we *make time* for ourselves (our whole self, with all its essential needs), there will never *be time* for ourselves.

If we think we do not have time to take care of ourselves now, how will we be able to recover from complete mental and psychological collapse? This is what burnout leads to. We may ignore our own needs, but the shutting down of our undernourished systems will happen on its own if we don't take care of ourselves. It is much smarter to be proactive and be in control of how much of ourselves we make available now and to what things, so that we do not become *completely unavailable* due to a total collapse in functioning.

You might be surprised to hear that it takes more energy, time, and effort to *recover* from burnout than it does to *prevent* it. Think of this as the gas tank in your car. You fill up the tank proactively as opposed to only when you can't drive anywhere any longer because you completely ran out. Running your car on empty can damage it and require expensive repairs. I wish we could see our needs in a similar manner and not try to restore our energy only when we are completely depleted, because it takes an enormous effort and time to restore ourselves back to baseline.

- As with most problems, it is easier to prevent them than to try and fix them once they occur.

So what could we do to prevent burnout? The way to begin is, first and foremost, with a change in perspective. We must have a clear understanding and an unconditional acceptance of our own significance as a person.

As selfless and ever-giving we may be, we must learn to see ourselves as our own most important resource. When we are depleted, we cannot fill up others. So step one is to really take time to acknowledge our human nature, our needs and desires, and give ourselves the permission to be taken care of. We must not only meet our needs on a regular basis, but also protect our resources. In other words, we have to set boundaries about *what* we can give, *when*, to *whom*, and *how much*. We will talk more about boundaries in the next chapter.

The bottom line is that once we see ourselves as whole, complex, nuanced human beings, we will see more than just our physical needs. And when we acknowledge our own importance, we will attend to the whole spectrum of our needs, not just the needs of the body. And when I say *acknowledge our own importance*, I do not mean that we do this in an arrogant at-others-expense kind of way. No-no. We do this in a responsible self-affirming way. The kind of way we discussed in Chapter 5.

You see, lack of life enjoyment and poor sense of wellbeing is not a result of some vague and currently disputed "chemical imbalance" that must be "corrected" with pharmaceutical interventions. Rather, it stems from *life imbalance* and neglected needs. While some painful emotions may be so debilitating that they may require such interventions in order to bring an individual back to a baseline of some minimum functioning capacity, it is never the full answer. Although medication may alleviate the distress we feel, it does not help us understand our emotions and the needs behind them, nor does it give us clues on how to meet them. That's why it is not the real answer. The real answer lies in understanding our needs and meeting them, one at a time. The good thing is that we have clear pointers as to *what* to pay attention to and *when* — because our emotions tell us so.

If you find yourself at a stage of burnout, individualized professional support can be really helpful. However, if you are able to turn things around before they begin to roll downhill, here are some suggestions that you can benefit from right away, as long as you implement them consistently.

The first suggestion I will make has to do with guilt.

We have to let it go. We will talk more about this in the next chapter (see section "Resolving Judgement and Guilt"). There is no place for guilt when it comes to taking care of oneself. You can think of guilt as something coming from those unhealthy beliefs we discussed at the beginning of this chapter. Also know that feeling guilty takes up time, brain space, and other resources from our already limited mental capacity. So if we spend time feeling guilty, it will further deplete our already compromised resources. If we are going to make space for something, let it be for the things that fill us up and are actually helpful, and not the ones that drain us even further.

The next thing you can do is an inventory of your needs.

You do this to find which ones are easier to meet and what gives you the most energy when you attend to them. And then be more intentional about making space for meeting those needs. It may be easier to start with the Core Need of Fun & Enjoyment. If you find that you really enjoy a solo walk in nature, that it really fills you up and you can usually get yourself out of the house for 20 minutes, then become proactive about making space for it.

Keep looking. What fills you up? What lights you up? What relaxes you and makes you feel at peace? Think about your answers and create small moments of nurture spread throughout the day (e.g., a page from your favorite book, a cup of delicious tea, a hobby, tinkering with things, and so on). Try to find a variety of activities, big and small, that bring you joy, make you smile, fill your cup, and restore your energy. Even a few minutes here and there dedicated to taking care of yourself will set the stage for managing the rest of the demands that your day brings that much better. When we make room for those smaller changes, we will see other opportunities and find new resources to do even more.

Truly make an effort to create space in your day for what fills you up.

Schedule time. Be intentional about it.

Spending time doing what you enjoy is not a luxury. It is a necessity.

To think that we do not have time for our needs is a deceptive story we tell ourselves that steals energy from our life. If you have time to mindlessly browse on your phone or computer, then you do have time to carve out for yourself. While social media and other mindless activities on our gadgets may give us a sense of a "quick fix," they are not designed to fill you up. Quite the opposite. They are designed to keep you *wanting more*, so you stick around, doing more of what does not serve you. Gadgets will not give you what your higher being really needs. So choose instead what will.

If you are not sure what lights you up, consider writing and reflecting about your feelings, thoughts, and reactions, as well as your aspirations and desires. Though writing may not be for everyone, it can be a powerful strategy to process some of our mind's resources that we otherwise may not have direct access to. Once you start writing, you might actually be surprised by the depth of your own thoughts and ideas. Afterall, when we make ourselves at the service of other people, we forget our own human side of being a real person, with real interests, passions, and needs.

Another thing you can do to prevent burnout is to examine your priorities and expectations. Not only will this help with some of the guilt you may be feeling, but it will also help you manage things differently.

Ask yourself, what is the absolute *must*? What *has* to happen, and what is a nice-to-have and can wait? It is amazing how many things we commit to without giving it a second thought. These "obligations" fill up our schedules but leave us empty inside. So think about it, what taxing and time-consuming routines can be changed or eliminated from your life? Perhaps temporarily, at least for now.

Assess what is reasonable to expect now, given how much you are juggling. If you were cooking an elaborate meal three times a day, what changes can you make to save a little bit more time for yourself? Now, if cooking is your joy and it is something that fills you up, you would be wise to keep that and cut down on something else. The point is, you are looking for opportunities to replace draining commitments and simplify your life so that there is more space in your life *for you*.

And finally, ask yourself whether you are living according to your own standards and expectations, or trying to meet someone else's. If it is your own expectations you are not living up to and are draining yourself in the process, would it make sense to modify those expectations to meet the reality of your life in the present moment?

Start thinking about these things.

There is always an answer. And if you want to hear more about managing expectations and dealing with guilt, we talk about that in the last chapter.

Chapter 8

Building Capacity For More

In this chapter, we will talk about increasing our capacity to meet our needs. Expanding our ability to fulfill our own needs means — having more resources. But not just *any* resources, we want to strive for better resources, the ones that are a good match for our needs.

Let's remember that simply expanding our bank of resources is not enough. In order for those additional resources to work well for us, we have to have two other components in place. And these are: *need awareness*, so that we know *which* resources will match our needs, and *emotion awareness,* so that we know *when* to deploy those resources and notice that they are called upon. The point is not to have more for the sake of having more, but to have an increased *ability* to respond to life demands and our ongoing needs in a timely manner. And so, although in this chapter we will focus more on the expansion of your options for resources, these two steps — emotion awareness and need awareness — are critical components to the full 3-Step Needs-Based Process and help make sure you are getting the results you want.

Before we explore additional areas to consider when looking for resources and ways to meet our needs, here is what I'd like you to keep in mind. When we want *more* of something, we can either *add* more or we can make sure we are *not losing* or wasting what we already have. Sometimes we expand our capacity by expanding our resources and actively looking for how to meet our needs in a new/better/more efficient way. And at other times, the way we make sure we have resources to meet our needs is by preserving whatever resources we *already have*. We do that by being more intentional about protecting them against unnecessary losses. When it comes to resources, there are definitely "holes" we can plug to prevent wasteful leaks. These are the different places in our lives where resources are being drained or are not properly utilized.

There are certain factors in our lives — people, places, and things — that tend to put undue strain on us, deplete our resources, and drain our energy. We can say that they *leak* our resources. Being aware of them helps us manage them better and determine how much of ourselves should be invested there.

We may also find that some of these things do not even need to be in our lives anymore, as they don't give anything back to us, waste our time and energy, and take up space in our mind. A good analogy to illustrate this concept is energy leaks in winter when the heat escapes through windows, doors, and so on. Obviously, we don't want to seal ourselves so tightly that we don't ever interact with the outside world (just like you wouldn't want to be unable to open a window or a door). On the contrary, we do want energy to flow, to be able to exchange resources with others. At the same time, we also want to be mindful and in control of our resources and where that energy goes.

So let's look at how to preserve what we have, so that we can have more of what we need.

MANAGING EXPECTATIONS

Expectations — especially unmet expectations — tend to occupy a lot of our mental space and, as such, can drain a lot of our mental resources. So let's talk about holding appropriate expectations for yourself and others when it comes to your needs.

First of all, let me tell you that we will not have *all* of our needs met, all at *once*, at *all* times. And it is not necessary. Meeting our needs is a dynamic and ongoing process. Some of our needs may be met partially and not completely, and that is OK too. Make a note of that and keep seeking additional resources. For example, we may have wanted to spend a whole day with a friend, but plans changed and we only saw them for a couple of hours. That's OK, as we can make the best of our time together and seek more opportunities like that in the future. Let's say we wanted to finish a book because it was so engaging and we wanted to know how it ends, but all we could get to was only a few pages. That's OK too. There is no reason to dismiss however little time we did get to spend with the book, and we can seek more opportunities to finish the rest of it later.

You can also expect that things that used to work well for you in the past, may not work as well now. You see, some of our needs shift and change as we mature and continue to develop personally. What used to be fun may not be fun anymore, or what used to matter no longer does. And that, too, is OK. In fact, my hunch is that we are designed this way. Meaning, as soon as all of our needs are met, it's an opportunity for us to seek new areas to evolve into, to stretch, and to grow. And so, when something within us changes and we have new pursuits to follow, this inevitably leads to changes in our needs.

Staying flexible, open minded, and curious is the best way to approach our changing and evolving needs. Say you used to enjoy alone time with a book, but now a book doesn't draw you in or you just don't feel like reading anymore. You can get curious and ask yourself, what other activity/resource would you prefer and feel drawn to, which would meet the same need that reading a book did? This, in turn, helps you get curious about which need was fulfilled through reading.

Some people read for the fun of it and some — in search of deeper meaning. For some, it is a way to rest and spend some time in solitude and quiet, whereas for others — it is a way to get information and make progress on something they are working on. What is it *for you*?

What alternative resource can meet the same need for you if reading no longer does? And even if you are not sure, being flexible and trying things out, will give you the answer eventually.

By adopting a "try it and see" approach, not only will you figure out what the need is, but you will also discover some good resources to meet that need. Make this approach your modus operandi, which is especially useful when things around us and within us are shifting, which is — all the time!

Even though a particular need may not be satisfied for some time, it is not a *neglected* need, because we are actively engaged with it and are considering different answers. All of this is to say that unmet needs are part of life's ebb and flow, and something you can expect to happen. And as long as we *strive* for balance and have the *majority* of our needs met, life will definitely feel satisfying and meaningful. On the other hand, when most of our needs are unmet, life can feel like a burden. And when life feels like a burden, we may begin to have unreasonable expectations, such as — expecting someone else to make it lighter. When we expect others to tend to our needs, we run the risk of becoming a burden to them.

An unexpected outcome of placing our needs in the hands of other people is that we may actually delay their satisfaction. For example, it is so much easier to get a glass of water myself, than to wait for someone else to do it for me. If, for some reason, I do have to rely on someone else to give me water, that does delay the answer to my need. If I am capable of meeting my needs, I shouldn't be expecting other to do it for me.

You see, even though we may have expectations for other people and their resources, we actually do not have any control over them. And that is what makes our expectations unreasonable, and obtaining resources this way — more taxing and unlikely to be successful. What also tends to happen when we expect others to take care of our needs is that, while we wait for them to do that, we are missing out on the opportunity to meet our needs on our own. Not only are we likely to get there faster, there is also a higher likelihood that we get our needs met exactly the way that suits us. For example, only I know how much water I need, and so I can pour myself the exact amount. Only I know how hot I want my tea to be, and so I can take care of that too, to perfection if I want to.

I always found it a bit humorous how a child may be asking an adult whose hands are busy with something to get a toy for them that they are perfectly capable of reaching themselves. And since they have to wait until the adult gets the toy for them, they begin to tantrum about it taking too long. Of course, I get it and have all the compassion for the child, because children are still learning about their own abilities and are still developing their sense of agency. But so many adults do this too! Instead of helping ourselves, we throw our own version of a tantrum when others aren't fast enough to drop what they are doing and come serve us.

This is a good place to remind ourselves that the 8 Core Psychological Needs that we reviewed in Chapter 5 are basic for a reason. Precisely because they are critical to our wellbeing, they are also relatively simple to meet *on our own*.

All we have to do is to develop better awareness around them and understand them. We make this process overly and unnecessarily complicated when we give it to other people and make them responsible for the job that isn't theirs to begin with. We need to realize that it takes more energy to "convince" other people to meet our needs, than it does to meet them on our own.

It may be the case that this assumption — of being dependent on others to meet our needs and of not being capable to satisfy our needs without their help — originated during the early stages in our development at a time when our psyche, the Self, was just beginning to be formed. You see, in early childhood, in order for the Self to be formed, someone else has to be there to meet its needs. And so just like the parent was responsible for meeting the child's *physical* needs, they did so for the child's *psychological* needs as well. Some parents did that better than others, but that's besides the point. The point is that this reliance on the "Other" to meet the needs of the "Self" is only natural in childhood, while the child is still dependent on adults for survival.

However, for a healthy psyche — the one that has been developmentally appropriately formed — that process of meeting one's own needs transfers onto the person themselves. Now that they can satisfy their *physical* needs independently of others, they should be able to do that for their *psychological* needs as well. And this makes sense because, if our survival truly depends on something, we should naturally have the capacity to take care of that ourselves. And when it comes to our needs, we do. So all of this is to say that, even though the Self depends on another person *initially* during its formation, it relies on *itself* for maintenance.

Just because we started out being taken care of by others, does not mean that it should continue this way or that it is natural to continue to rely on that. To expect from others and to depend on others is counter to the basic principles of autonomy, which is key to evolution, vitality, and survival.

The idea of attending to your needs yourself, as opposed to waiting on others to meet your needs for you, isn't new. In her quite famous book, "Codependent No More," Melody Beattie warns that: "'The surest way to make ourselves crazy is to get involved with other people's businesses, and the quickest way to become sane and happy is to tend to our own affairs." An alcoholic by the time she graduated high school, Beattie spoke from years of experience in codependent relationships. She suffered the dysfunction of depending on someone else for years, until she decided to take care of herself and find what she needed.

- Expecting that other people will meet our needs, often leads to disappointment.

If others know exactly what we need and are able to provide it — wonderful! You've got yourself an extra resource. But when they don't, which is often the case (because other people are wise to attend to their own needs first), we should have plenty of skills and an arsenal of resources to be able to meet our needs on our own.

The disappointment that we experience (which, by the way, lands within the continuum of Sadness) speaks to the loss of expected resources. We were hoping and expecting that others will do something to meet our needs. When they don't, that assumed resource goes away and is experienced as a loss.

If we help someone, expecting them to meet our needs in return, we may feel indignant (which is a feeling within the Anger continuum) when they don't. We may feel it is unfair and then try to control others in an attempt to make sure that they return the favor. But I hope you and I can agree what a waste of time and resources that is! Attempting to control other people consumes so much more energy than it does to simply take control over our own life, our own needs, and our own actions.

So since we are talking about depending on other people, let's check in with ourselves... Is this happening to you? Given that one of the reasons why people have a hard time meeting their needs is because they make themselves dependent on others, it is important to check ourselves. In our society, there is a lot of confusion in regards to the responsibilities and roles people have when it comes to needs, which leads many of us to associate needs and their satisfaction with relationships.

Consequently, this creates an impression that satisfaction of our needs depends on the quality of our relationships with other people, and so relationships with others are being prioritized at the expense of our relationship with ourselves. Just think about how many times you have said *"no" to yourself* so that you can say *"yes" to others*? And how many times has it happened that you said yes, even though it was against your values, just to appease others, be liked or be approved of, or maybe so that in the future others return the favor and attend to your needs? All of that erodes our relationship with ourselves and gets in the way of getting our needs met.

The reverse of this is not only more appropriate, it is also more effective.

Meaning, the quality of our life truly depends on the quality of attention we give to ourselves and the extent to which our needs are met. If we make the quality of our life dependent on our relationships with others, we may end up chasing the wrong things, pursuing people, wasting time appeasing them, and so on, instead of investing time and resources in taking care of ourselves. Making our needs our own priority and responsibility not only improves our relationship with ourselves, but also — with others. Why? Because we no longer put the pressure of our expectations onto other people and do not make it their burden to meet our needs. However, if we do the opposite, we put ourselves at risk for codependent relationship dynamics.

If you place the responsibility for your needs on you — then the quality of your life depends on you. If you place it on others — it will depend on others. If we understand that we have little to no control over others, we can also see why it is so frustrating when we decide to put our needs in the hands of other people. When, however, we gain full control and responsibility over our needs — our quality of life not only increases, it is in our full control. And that, in turn, reinforces our Sense of Agency. Managing expectations appropriately, builds our capacity to do more for ourselves. And since it is our job to meet our needs, why wait?

MEETING NEEDS PROACTIVELY

Being in control of our needs helps us be proactive in attending to them. Unmet needs and needs that go unattended for a while begin to "nag" at us, and that "nagging" can start to drain our energy. This is the reason why when we meet needs on time or as soon as we can (to the best of our ability, of course), we free up additional resources.

This may sound a bit counterintuitive at first. If we need resources to meet our needs, then how do we get to have more resources? This happens because when needs are met, they become a resource by means of giving us more energy, more vitality, more capacity to do other things.

- When our needs are not met they will *require* resources.

- But as soon as they are met they *become* a resource.

Since satisfied needs have this ability to give us "life energy" and support our wellbeing, it would only make sense to have access to this resource sooner rather than later. And that is why meeting our needs proactively as they arise (as opposed to waiting until they start draining us), is a wise thing to do.

This may be easier to grasp if we use an example of a physical need. If we are hungry, this sensation of an unmet need will interfere with our ability to do other things. Taking a moment to satisfy this need may slow us down initially, but once it's met, it will give us even more energy and fuel our capacity for more. And that makes it even more possible for us to access additional resources and meet other needs of ours going forward.

Now, imagine not pausing to take a moment to take care of that need. Would it go away? Nope. It will begin to nag and interfere with our ability to move on with our day. The fact that we are satiated, means we are now more able to do the next thing, as opposed to feeling depleted and unable to think of anything besides finding something to eat. In a similar fashion, when we find our work meaningful (i.e., our need for meaning and purpose is satisfied), it gives us motivation and drive. Both of these are great energetic resources, which help us do the work even when it is hard. Or, when the need for rest is met, that fulfilled need becomes a resource, because now we have energy to focus on whatever is in front of us.

Although, as previously discussed, it is highly unlikely that we will have all of our needs met at all times, it helps to be proactive as much as we can so that there is a comfortable balance between met and unmet needs. Too many unmet needs will tip the scale and turn them into overwhelm and stress. The more unmet needs we carry, the less likely we are to be able to fulfill them. It's like trying to juggle too many things. If we find ourselves in such a situation, we have to begin to prioritize or find a temporary compromise in terms of which resources we tap into in order to satisfy our needs, at least at the very basic level, if not fully.

- The fewer unmet and neglected needs we have, the more likely it is that the needs that do come up will be attended to in a timely manner.

"Timely" is really the word to pay attention to. Not only does that prevent burnout, which we talked about in the previous chapter, but it arms you with the right kind of attitude. The kind of attitude that says — you matter and your needs matter. The right attitude about this also helps you set boundaries around your needs and your resources (more on that in the next section of this chapter). It puts you in the best position to handle your day. Imagine what would happen if before you go on a trip of several hundred miles, you don't make sure your tank is full? Yeah, you won't get far.

And what if you decided to put only a gallon of gas every time you needed to pull into a gas station? Yup, that would not be a reasonable way to manage your energy and resources.

Meeting needs proactively, will make you better prepared to face various challenges, from minor hiccups to more demanding life situations. There will be times when immediate fulfillment of your needs may not be possible and so it would serve you best if you arrive at those times generally taken care of, as opposed to — already depleted. It will give you confidence, resilience, and the ability to wait until new resources become available to you. It will grow your capacity to handle life demands. Also, if you generally have a habit of meeting your needs, you will not miss the opportunity to do so, when that opportunity presents itself. You will attend to your needs as soon as possible, because of a habit of doing it.

We owe it to ourselves to put ourselves first.

That is the only way we can be available to others.

If we are having trouble with the concept of putting ourselves first, burnout will eventually let itself be known. Our attitude needs to align with our aspirations, so that it drives our actions. When other people's needs are always a priority, we never receive the time, care, and attention that we also need. When we think that we can wait and just have to muster up some more strength and courage and simply push ourselves to continue, we actually make our lives that much harder.

Oh, but what if you simply don't have time for your needs? The reality is that we find time for the things that matter. As I mentioned before, it takes less time to attend to your needs, than it does to deal with all the stress and heartache that unmet needs result in. Taking yourself seriously and attending to your needs is a priority for which you should *make the time.*

We can only do more if we have capacity for more.

Increasing our capacity is in our hands.

RESOLVING JUDGMENT & GUILT

Before we can talk more specifically about *where* and *how* to find more resources, we have to address a major issue, a black hole of sorts that will suck in all of your resources — current and future ones — no matter how many you've got or will try to acquire. Remember, whatever can take an inch, can also take a mile, and it will take that mile inch by inch. You won't even notice. Except, you will be left wondering why you are feeling so depleted all the time. We want to prevent that from happening. There shouldn't be any black holes that suck your energy and resources without your awareness and permission.

One such big black hole is guilt.

Another one is — other people's judgments about us.

Usually these two feed each other, because guilt has its roots in other people's judgments about us, real or perceived. The conversation we just had at the beginning of this chapter about releasing expectations that *we* have for other people is very relevant here. We also talked about Self vs. Other, when it comes to who is responsible for our needs. And those principles go both ways. In other words, when it comes to meeting our needs, not only do we drop expectations *of* others, we also do not accept expectations *from* them.

Our needs are *our* responsibility.

Other people's needs are *their* responsibility.

Just like us, other people have the ability and the potential to meet their needs, do their best to understand what works for them, and find resources they need in order to meet them. Each one of us, even if currently we may not feel like we have what's required to meet our needs, can and will find a way, as long as we take responsibility for them. And just as we are not responsible for other people's needs, we are not accountable to their judgments and expectations.

Really, think about it. What exactly is the point of trying to get approval from people, especially the one you don't even like anyway?

Those who truly depend on us (e.g., little children, elderly, and sick family members) are, of course, our responsibility, but even then it would not be wise to attend to their needs at our own expense. Of course there are emergencies. There will be times you drop everything and rush to care for someone else. However, I must caution you against making this a habit. We don't want to be living our lives as if in a constant state of emergency. Yet, so many of us do that!

Now, there will always be people *who think* they depend on us and would love for us to share this belief with them so that we help them meet their needs. We have to be able to tell the difference between those who are truly unable to take care of themselves and those who are perfectly capable but would rather other people do it for them. The latter group will always have judgments about us, complaining and pouting that we don't do enough for them, don't give them enough of our time, energy, attention, and other resources. They are easy to spot because they try to make you feel guilty when you are choosing to attend to yourself and your needs.

So when we do engage with these kinds of people, we must ask ourselves, are we doing that because we truly want to *and* have the capacity for, or are we doing it out of guilt? Even when we want to, we have to be aware that there is a difference between *enabling dependence* (which is the kind of help that is getting in the way of people's ability to take care of themselves) and *facilitating independence* (which is all about helping people help themselves).

One is disempowering and the other — empowering.

And when we do have dependents, this is when we need to be especially diligent about meeting our own needs, and being proactive about that. Why? Because we are faced with even more demands that tap into our resources. So we have to make sure we are replenishing those resources on a regular basis, because not only do we have to meet our own needs, we've got to have extra reserves in order to help those who truly depend on us. Not only do we take care of another, we also must take care of ourselves. And you already know in what order that needs to happen. You come first.

But what about guilt?

Guilt shows up when you hold yourself accountable to someone else's standard, to someone else's expectations, even though deep down you don't want to. And it so happens that a lot of the things we feel guilt about are not even in our control.

Feeling responsibility and guilt for things that are neither your responsibility nor in your control is the most self-destructive and toxic feeling you can have. And because it has nothing to do with your own needs, you have to learn to release it. It is worth pointing out that guilt is often confused with remorse, and so I want to make sure you understand the difference. Remorse is a very different feeling and one that has deep personal meaning to us. For that reason, we will talk more about remorse in Chapter 10 because it is something we do want to pay attention to.

But guilt is not the kind of emotion we want to carry with us. It is an emotional trap. There is no answer to it, no way to get out, because it isn't our needs and expectations we are dealing with but someone else's. And oftentimes it is not even clear who is behind them and what exactly they want from us. I am talking about both, those individuals that never tell you what they want and expect you to guess and serve them, as well as those vague traditional or cultural expectations that have no face, yet feel so oppressive.

Since it is unclear where the expectation is coming from, it can be hard to pinpoint if we feel guilt because we *did* something, we *think* we did something, or we *failed* to do something. And so we resort to general people-pleasing, just in case, secretly hoping it will earn us "extra points" in advance of those people judging us.

If you've done this, no judgment here. We all have.

This is a lesson we learn after we realize that there is no end to the guilt game no matter how much we please others or how much we give in at our own expense. Not to mention that when we are just beginning to learn about our needs, we all make mistakes in how we allocate our resources. It's all part of the learning-about-ourselves process. It is mistakes like these that let us know how depleting people-pleasing is, how ineffective it is in attempting to resolve guilt, and how empty it leaves you.

And when we reach that point, of feeling empty, of nothing more to give, another feeling takes hold and that is — resentment. Resentment is a strong emotional signal we really should pay attention to because it speaks to us about neglected needs of our own.

Resentment is part of the Anger continuum and, as we discussed in Chapter 4, anger is a basic emotion. Like all basic negative emotions, it is telling us that something is not right. When it comes to anger, and resentment in particular, the message it is sending us is that something is unjust and not fair. Of course it's unfair.

- Our feelings are never wrong.

Since our emotions speak to our needs, what we feel is never wrong, because our needs are never wrong. So when we people-please and choose to act out of guilt, we deny ourselves. And that — is wrong. When we neglect ourselves, we neglect what we are directly responsible for — our needs. And that is not fair. No wonder why you would feel resentment.

- The feeling of resentment is *the sign* that you are not nurturing yourself enough.
- It is *the sign* that you need to do something about your mixed-up priorities.

Yes, we have a responsibility towards those who depend on us and we do feel called to help others, but we are also responsible for ourselves. If you ever wondered why you are so angry or resentful, guilt may be the reason. As counterintuitive as it sounds at first, the more guilt we carry and the more we do for others, the more likely we are to get resentful. This happens because when we act out of guilt, we act at our own expense (giving others what we ought to give to ourselves), and deep down we realize that this isn't fair.

Resentment is a natural delayed response to guilt and here is why. When we take on the burden of guilt, it is as if we are asked to take responsibility that is not *ours* to take on or that we don't *want* to carry but feel forced to. And so it is natural to have a sense of resistance rise up inside us. That resistance moves to defensiveness, then transforms into resentment, and then anger. It is like being brought to court for the crimes you have not committed, to defend yourself against the standards that weren't yours to begin with.

It doesn't feel fair, and it isn't.

The only way we can genuinely help others without expecting anything in return, is when we are called to do so from our heart. And that only happens when our heart is full and ready to give. Never at our own expense. And not from a sense of obligation.

When guilt is what drives our decisions, as opposed to our own needs and values, we end up feeling used and taken advantage of. When we allow ourselves to be taken advantage of, we are more likely to feel victimized and, when we act like a victim, we lose our perspective on how many things are actually in our control. However, when we take responsibility for things that are in our control, we increase our capacity to show up as our best selves. And that inevitably leads to better support for ourselves and an increased ability to support others when we feel inclined to.

So how do we not get deceived?

How do we avoid feeling like a victim?

We watch out for guilt. It is not an emotion in the Basic Triad of Discomfort (which consists of Anger, Sadness, and Fear), and so it speaks against our needs and not on our behalf. It sets up an unfair dynamic from the get go. You see, when negative emotions come up — any one from the Basic Triad of Discomfort — we know to look for a need we must attend to. It is pretty straightforward.

Conversely, when we are consumed by thoughts and ruminations that accompany guilt, we do not have answers and it is not clear as to what we should do. Since the feeling of guilt feels like harassment, we want to get rid of it as soon as we can, and so we may act impulsively to appease, thus losing sight of what is important to us. In service of silencing the guilt we may compromise on our own values.

In the short term — when we act driven by guilt — we may feel relief, but in the long-term — we lose.

When we lose, others we care about lose too. How? When we feel down and depleted, angry or resentful, others we love don't get the best of us.

Releasing people's expectations does not mean ignoring those people. It means having a choice. We can choose to only attend to those we care about (what a relief, eh?) or those whom we feel a mutual connection with. Life is short, resources take time and effort to acquire, and it is not our responsibility to serve everyone, especially at our own expense. And if your needs are not met while you are attending to others — you *are* doing it at your own expense, just so we are clear.

When we are talking about releasing guilt and not caring about other people's judgments, we are not talking about having no empathy and lacking understanding for what others may need. Freeing ourselves from guilt does not free us from the responsibility to do the best we can for those *in our care*. Quite the opposite. It gives us space to attend to our responsibilities, by letting go of what is *not* our responsibility.

Society does not have a place in dictating our priorities, only we do.

It makes suggestions and promotes agendas, but ultimately we decide what matters to us.

When we know ourselves, our values, and our own needs, we will put them first. When we don't, we end up following others who do. When we become disconnected and unable to nurture ourselves, that is when we invite other voices to tell us what they think we need and we allow for others to decide on our behalf.

Anyone can make a request and seek our resources and attention. Any person or organization can ask you to donate your time, money, attention, etc. Anyone can have an expectation on how much others (ourselves included) "owe" them. And yet, it is up to us how we interpret those requests and expectations.

Are they in alignment with what is important to us? To what extent are we willing and able to support others and respond to their requests (even when they come from those who depend on you, like your children)? And these are not the questions that the people making requests should be answering. They don't know your needs, values, responsibilities, and resources. Only you do. Even if they think they know, they are not you, and so all they can do is make assumptions. These are the questions to ask *yourself*, because the answers to them are within you. And when you know your answer, setting boundaries about what matters becomes so much easier.

ESTABLISHING BOUNDARIES

It is absolutely critical to have boundaries around your resources. Not having them is a sure way to drain your capacity to attend to your needs and the needs of those you care about. I know we've said this before, but it is quite important that we don't forget this point. What we talked about in the previous segment of this chapter — releasing guilt and expectations — is the starting point to establishing boundaries and protecting our resources.

When we have no boundaries, we may become a free-for-all resource for others without intending to and not even be aware of it. That will result in resource "leaks." Having boundaries allows you to preserve what works for you and to prevent unnecessary losses in your resources, so that you don't find yourself asking things like "Where did all of my time go?" or "Why do I feel so drained all the time?"

Of course, it goes without saying that helping others, being a resource to them, and being of service is a noble and meaningful pursuit. But only if done properly.

What this means is that it's not done at our own expense (e.g., meeting the needs of others ahead of our own) and that it is not done at the other people's expense either (e.g., doing things that others can do for themselves, like spoon-feeding a 10-year old child). We must have healthy boundaries when it comes to our resources and use our own discernment to be able to tell whether we are allowing others to take advantage of us. Sharing our resources and doing things for others is only going to work in healthy relationships that are balanced, reciprocal, and fair. The minute they are not, it becomes a drain on our resources, a gaping hole we can only close by changing the dynamics of that relationship.

Speaking of dynamics, I find them amazing in so many ways. There are various natural laws that govern how things work in the natural world and influence the dynamics of human relationships. There are laws of physics, there are laws of human nature, and there are principles behind everything that functions in the universe (including why we have needs in the first place and how they show up). One of the amazing ways in which these natural laws work is that they provide resources to those who need them.

Those who seek, do find.

And those who disregard, lose.

This means that there are always resources out there to meet our basic needs. If we are struggling to see them, it has more to do with our limited awareness of what our needs are and what/where/how resources may be available, than it does with whether resources are out there. This is such an important principle to understand. Meaning, that naturally — by the very nature of who we are and by the nature of our design — resources are available for our core needs. And our very nature makes sure we find them. We even have the greatest navigational tools that help us find what we need and they come in the form of our basic emotions. That is why we are still here, functioning, living, making it work. However perfectly or imperfectly we are able to do that is besides the point at the moment. The point is — there are always resources available.

And if you follow this principle all the way through, you may realize that what this also means is that *underutilized* resources turn into *available* resources for someone else, and will naturally flow to those who need them. And so if you are: a) not claiming resources, b) not using your resources, and c) not protecting them... what do you think will happen? Those resources will flow to those who seek them and need them.

That is why when our cup is full, we are naturally and instinctively inclined to help others, because we may have an excess of resources at that moment. At the same time, this principle also means the following:

- Other people will find your underutilized resources and will claim them.

Anything you are undervaluing and underutilizing becomes a resource signal for others. In other words, if you are underutilizing your time, other people will take it. If you are undervaluing your skills, other people will take advantage of them. If you are not protecting your thinking and are not making space in your mind for what matters to you, other people's ideas, thoughts, and beliefs will take space there.

I want to make sure you are hearing me right. This isn't about blaming other people or getting angry at them for claiming what you consider to be yours. That's not the proper perspective. What I am talking about here is a matter of a natural dynamic, a natural law of resources. You either claim a resource and you use it, or it naturally "wants" to go to someone else who will. So if you feel like you need something and it is your right to have, all you must be mindful of is whether you are using it, and whether you are respecting and protecting it. And that is what the concept of boundaries around our resources is all about.

The reason why we release other people's judgments and expectations of us, as we said in the previous segment, is because it has to do with them and their needs. And it really helps to understand that *the reason* they have judgments and expectations is because they are seeking resources for their needs, just like you are. It's just that they are going about it in the wrong way. Meaning, they are looking at others to meet their needs instead of looking at themselves. So the way to communicate to them that your resources are not available to them (unless you so intentionally choose), is to: a) release their judgments and expectations as having no importance to you and b) set boundaries around what's yours.

The best way you can help yourself to set boundaries is by reminding yourself of your value and importance as a worthy human being, and then by acting from your values, from a place of integrity. Boundaries is the line in the sand, so to speak, that says — this is mine and that is yours. When it comes to our needs, it is the line that says — these are my needs and my responsibility, and those are other people's needs and their responsibility. Likewise, when it comes to resources, we respect our own and other people's boundaries by drawing the line between our resources and other people's resources.

You can think of boundaries as rules you have for yourself.

These rules articulate what you will and will not allow.

It is a set of rules you live by that helps you protect your resources, and in doing so — protect your needs. It is what helps you decide when you say to others "Yes, I would love to" and "No, I won't be able to" or when to say "Yes, this works for me" and "No, that does not work for me."

What needs of yours are met before you meet the needs of others is your decision. You decide and you are in control. The only person who would know if your boundary is right or not — is you. If you are not sure your boundary is the right one for you, look for clues in signs of resentment. Resentment will show itself when we are not attending to our needs, which would mean that our boundary is too loose. Resentment tells us what it is we have not done for ourselves and reminds us to stop ignoring core needs of our own. In a way, resentment is an inverse of guilt. And, in this case, it can be seen as equivalent to feeling guilt for not taking care of ourselves (as opposed to feeling guilty for not taking care of others).

It is not up to random people to set our boundaries and remind us of our own needs. It is our job. Everyone around us has needs and will seek different ways of meeting them, including — seeing us as a resource to them, the source of their solution. We are the ones deciding whether that aligns with our priorities or not, and whether we have capacity for that or not.

- When we force ourselves into doing what we truly do not want to do, we violate our own boundaries.

When we so easily disrespect what is important to us, it compromises our ability to meet our needs. When we force ourselves to serve others out of obligation, we end up feeling justified to force others as well into something they are not comfortable with. And that, of course, is not fair to them.

In appeasing others, we may forget what priorities and needs we have. We may even interpret other people's needs as our own, and that is definitely a conflict of boundaries. Or, we may delegate our own authority by assuming that someone else knows best, and we may switch places and let others control the situation by placing their needs above our own needs and values.

Good boundaries, on the other hand, will help us understand that other people's feelings, needs, and beliefs are their own. Everyone is responsible for their own needs and wants, feelings and thoughts, actions and behaviors.

Good boundaries protect us from resentment. Think about it... When we feel resentment, whatever the reason, if we reflect on the situation that got us there, we will see that, even though there was something we needed to do for ourselves, a priority for us personally, we instead did what someone else wanted. Even if that someone is our child, our friend, or a family member, we must listen to what is ok and not ok with us. When we don't do that, we are setting ourselves up for resentment. To prevent that, we really must honor our own needs, which will help us build good boundaries around them.

We protect what matters.

We look after what's ours.

If we don't protect it and we do not look after it, it is either because we have lost sight of what matters or have no ownership over what's ours. If a reminder is helpful here, let me say this again — your needs are yours, and they do matter. Your resources are yours and they are worth looking after. And when we miss that, we can bet our emotions will let us know we've wandered off the path of integrity.

HOLDING SPACE FOR GRATITUDE

I am holding my fingers crossed that you don't skip this section. The word "gratitude" has become so commonplace that it has lost its potency in communicating how powerful the concept itself is. When we skip gratitude, we miss out on a huge resource that can help us build our capacity to have even more resources.

When you say thank you for what you have, two special things happen (among other wonderful outcomes): you begin to notice what you already have and you become even more self-aware. Awareness of what we have and what we appreciate increases our awareness of what works for us and how we can have more of it. So gratitude sets off ripples that reach into new domains and help us find new/more resources. Gratitude is like saying: "Thank you. I would like some more of that please." It allows you to have what you need, because it helps you *see* what you need by appreciating what you have.

When you develop the awareness of what you are thankful for, your needs and what serves them becomes even more clear to you. That clarity allows you to pursue more of what works for you. Since gratitude is a source of positive emotions as well, in that way — it also becomes a resource. It is a reminder of where else your cup becomes full. It shows you which of your needs are met and how.

Now, this is not to be used to invalidate any *unmet* needs you may currently have.

People are often told to be grateful for what they have, as a means of curtailing additional needs and wishes. That is simply not right. This is how gratitude is often misused. What I am offering instead is to see in what ways your cup is full so that it can give you courage, hope, and even confidence to know that you will find a way to meet the rest of your needs as well. It helps you see that meeting your needs has happened before and, therefore, will happen again. Gratitude allows you to recognize and acknowledge that.

It is easy to forget how much we have in our lives, what we are deeply grateful for. It is easy to slip into negative thinking patterns and only see the dark side of things, the lack.

Gratitude keeps us in a balanced frame of mind to see opportunities where a negatively oriented mind will be too closed off to see them. We are not talking about the kind of idealistic positive thinking that borders on denial of your needs or your situation. I mean, the whole purpose of this book is to teach you how to become aware of your needs, to acknowledge the challenges, and to look for solutions. And so a realistic and solution-oriented attitude is more practical and helpful here than either of these two: idealistic positive thinking or, its opposite, pessimistic attitude of helplessness.

There are so many things we are thankful for, but in our hectic days we either forget to treasure them or take them for granted. We would know immediately how much they mean to us if, all of a sudden, we were to lose them. Well, what if I told you that by not being actively grateful for what we have, we *are slowly losing sight of it* and are making it less valuable and less available to us. So let's make sure that what we value and are grateful for helps us keep things in perspective.

Of course, it could always be worse, but that is not the reason why we want to be grateful. Rather, it is because it can be *even better*. But in order for it to be better, we need to acknowledge what is already working. This kind of perspective is often what's needed in order to help us take the right action or to see new opportunities and resources.

And while all of this is great, there are a couple of things I need to warn you about.

There may be a problem with gratitude, when we don't use this practice correctly. When we hold space for gratitude in our lives, we also must hold space for ourselves, which means that sometimes you are just not feeling grateful. Sometimes you will feel miserable and like nothing is working. So make sure to hold space for that instead of trying to ignore your feelings in order to shift into gratitude.

Don't try and "do gratitude" if it does not resonate with you in those moments. Don't force it. When we force ourselves into gratitude, we are least likely to benefit from it. Gratitude can only become a resource for you if it works for you as a practice. Otherwise, it becomes a meaningless mantra. This is true for any and all of our resources, as we have previously discussed. If something does not work for us or does not help us meet our needs, it is not the right resource for us at that moment. It only works if it works, not if you are *forcing* it to work.

Although the no-forcing approach is something that can be said about any strategies and resources we use to fulfill our needs, I feel that it is especially important to point this out when it comes to gratitude, because the practice of gratitude has become so mainstream that you may feel like you *have* to do it.

Gratitude seems to be the new "have-to," like flossing your teeth. However, even though now and then you may have to force yourself to floss your teeth, there is no point in forcing yourself into gratitude. Whereas your teeth will benefit from your efforts, no matter how you felt about it in the process, gratitude does not work like that. It is all about how you feel, and you cannot lie to yourself about how you feel. You may certainly try — and some of us do — but it doesn't get us anywhere.

If you have noticed, there is a theme in this book, and that is — *sincerity around what you feel.*

It's a private conversation between you and... you.

It will only *serve* you if you are honest with yourself. If you pretend you feel one thing and not another, you will misunderstand your needs and what to do to bring yourself back to balance. So if gratitude is not what you feel, then don't pretend you do. Your feelings and needs are between you and you. No one else would know if you are lying to yourself. But *you* certainly will. Don't do yourself a disservice.

Also, do not use gratitude against yourself.

Do not use gratitude as a way to be mean to yourself.

What am I talking about? So often we use gratitude as a stick to beat ourselves up. It's when we say things like "I should be grateful" or "How dare I ignore my blessings." Stop it. Don't do that. The reason you may not be able to hold space for gratitude is because you may need to hold space for yourself first. There is the right time and there is the wrong time. It is definitely the wrong time to force yourself into gratitude when what you really need is space for yourself.

- Gratitude is not a substitute for validation.

Sometimes what you really need is validation and acknowledgment of what you are going through and what you may be needing. To be seen, to be heard comes ahead of gratitude. Gratitude is the way to see what is working and to see *ourselves* in the context of what is working, to see which needs are met.

But the other side of seeing also has to be present. That means that we also need to be able to see when things are *not* working, are *not* there, *not* serving us, etc. It's a balance of both. And so sometimes what helps is for us to see ourselves inside the struggle we are in, to truly understand what we may be going through, and support ourselves through that with the tools of acknowledgment and validation. In other words, sometimes what we need most — is to give ourselves compassion, empathy, and understanding *for what is not well*, as opposed to only looking for *what is well*.

Understanding *what is not well* is also of service to us, because that is the way that we begin to see our needs, which then allows us to look for resources to meet them. And that is something to be grateful for as well — for our capacity to hold space for ourselves when we need it. So don't demand gratitude from yourself, when what you truly need is *to be seen* as you are, where you are, with all the challenges that you may be facing. Give yourself that acknowledgment. Validate what needs to be validated, hear what needs to be heard, and see what needs to be seen in you and for you.

And gratitude will come.

EXPANDING AWARENESS

Since the process of getting to a balanced life relies on these three qualities — emotion awareness, need awareness, and resource awareness, — then the way we build capacity for more is by intentionally expanding our awareness and knowledge in these three areas.

This is an intentional process that requires you to ask more and better questions, to look beyond what you already know, and be willing to put effort into learning more about yourself, your inner life, and the world around you. When you invest time and attention in getting to know yourself and your unique expression of needs, you will be better able to meet them, especially as they change and evolve alongside your own growth.

- When we find resources, we learn to see more of them.
- Awareness leads to more awareness.

This process happens naturally. Since our needs are so core to our survival as human beings (the whole essence of ourselves, not just our bodies), we will *naturally* be on the lookout for ways to meet them. That is a given. But we can also do this with *intention* by wanting to grow in our self-awareness.

The best way to start is by practicing the three steps of the Needs-Based Process on an ongoing basis and slowing down along the way to reflect on what we are learning about ourselves. Through this practice and by going through each of the three steps of this process intentionally, time and time again, we will begin to understand our needs better, as well as how our emotions communicate with us. When we pay close attention, we take notice of what resources work best for us. And when we see what's working, we can have more of it. It is only through practice that we can:

- expand our ability to detect discomfort and negative emotions
- expand our ability to understand the needs that have to be met
- expand our awareness of what resources are available to us

Each of these levels of awareness can expand even more when we intentionally ask questions and want to learn more about our emotions, our needs, and the ways in which to meet them. It's time to listen even more closely to yourself, your body, your mind.

Listen to hear your needs and to understand your values. In a very basic sense it boils down to the willingness to grow — to understand who you are, what drives you, what is meaningful to you, how the needs we discussed show up in your life, how they express you. When we grow, we naturally expand our reach, our resources, and our capacity to meet our needs. The more awareness we have, the more mindful we become about proactively meeting our needs, which is what helps us maintain internal sense of harmony and feel the undeniable sense of aliveness.

Any type of clutter in your life (mental, physical, relational, etc.) will drain you without this awareness. How? Because it is constantly calling your attention to it and preoccupies your mind. So get in the habit of asking: What can I let go of? What people, places, and things do not serve me anymore? What can I let go of so that I can free up space for myself and have the capacity for the kind of resources that do meet my needs? More questions to ask are:

- Is it giving you joy?
- Is it helpful in some way?
- Is it meaningful?
- Is it doing the job of serving you?

No, no, and no? Then it's gotta go. One of the skills that will help you here (remember that skills are resources too!) is saying no, saying goodbye, and setting boundaries.

Removing clutter from your life, ending engagements with things that are not working, and quieting the noise... All of that will create space for you to see opportunities and potential in the areas that do actually serve you. All of us have the capacity to tell what's not working. All we need for that is tune in to our emotions and be honest about what we are feeling.

In other words, as long as you put it into practice, your knowledge around the 3-Step Needs-Based Process will evolve into skills and capacities you may not currently have. As you get to know your needs, you may discover that there are additional resources — such as skills, qualities, opportunities, etc. — that you do not currently have. That's OK. Make a list of all of them and make it your goal to obtain them. These are the areas of opportunity and potential for more growth for you. And any growth and expansion we achieve will lead to more resources. When you make your list, prioritize internal over external areas of growth, because when we grow as individuals and expand our personal strengths, we can take them with us no matter where we go.

This quality makes internal resources the most reliable and accessible ones of them all.

This could be any number of things, like improving your overall health, developing strong values, expanding interpersonal skills, sharpening our reasoning and problem-solving abilities, and so on. It is beyond the scope of this book to show you step by step *how* to acquire each one of these resources. However, you can decide which ones are important to you, what you want to pursue, and focus your attention on seeking out additional information about the "how-to" of developing these resources even further.

I would not recommend pursuing *any* of these, however, without first resolving energy leaks and resource drains you may already be experiencing (the "black holes" we talked about in the previous section). Why? No matter what new resources you acquire, you will be unlikely to benefit from them, because they will escape you if you do things at your own expense. Many people also find that, once they've plugged in those "holes" of guilt or other people's judgments and expectations, they actually have enough resources to meet their needs without seeking new ways. So, before you go after new abilities and skills, I encourage you to start there first and revisit previous sections of this chapter if you need to.

Now, assuming you are making sure you are not wasting resources already available to you and do not have any "holes" that require your attention, here is another way you can expand your awareness of the kind of resources that may be available. To see what else is possible for us, we can get curious about the world. How do things work? What makes them work even better?

You can start by looking at other people you know (or, perhaps, even admire) and get curious about them. What is it they do that seems to work for them? How do they meet their needs? What qualities, characteristics, skills, resources do you see them use that you would love to have too. Make a list.

It is OK to also look at those aspects of other people's lives that you may be jealous or envious of. These emotions are signals that others have something you also would like to have and feel it is your right to have. Great! Add those things to the list as well.

- And then ask yourself, what do you need to do in order to acquire these resources?

Remember to test them as you go, to make sure these resources do indeed work for you, that they do meet your needs. Not everything that works for others will work for us. Trying things is how we can test our assumptions and predictions. And then we adopt what works and discard what doesn't.

Let's never forget that it isn't the tactics, the skills, or the tools that make a particular resource great, but its *fit* to our needs. So always strive for a resource/need match, as we discussed in Chapter 6.

Chapter 9

How Not To Process Emotions

Up to this point, we have focused on *what* to do with emotions and *how* to resolve emotional discomfort and distress. It is also important that we talk about *how not to* and things to avoid. As you continue to explore the world of emotions, you will come across various schools of thought. Some of them offer good tools and some, unfortunately, promote methods of emotional regulation that are not very helpful.

Given the nature of my work and the many years of professional practice, I have seen countless models and methods. Some of them are helpful, some don't work at all, while others only work if you work even harder. And so I would be remiss if I didn't mention them here. Of course, like everything else in this book, I leave it up to you to use your discernment and decide what works for you best.

If a particular method is calling to you, I invite you to try it (test it for fit, as we discussed in the previous chapter) and judge its effectiveness for yourself. You may find that certain aspects of other methods are attractive to you or useful in some way. Some of them may feel very helpful and complete in addressing your emotional experiences, but some — you will find — only work *to an extent* or only *somewhat*. If that is the case, then information offered in this chapter should help you figure out what may be missing in a particular method, so that you can add those missing links based on what we have discussed in this book.

In fact, you can test any method or model against the Three Steps in the Needs-Based Process, which I find are always necessary in order to achieve the full resolution to any emotional tension (as opposed to simply obtaining a temporary relief). Many helpful models invite you to attend to your emotions (Step 1), which is great, but this is only the beginning to living a balanced life and is not enough for a sustained sense of inner peace and vitality. To stay consistently in touch with our sense of aliveness, we have to also attend to our needs, not only our emotions. This is what I see missing in most other methods: a direct conversation about the needs (Step 2) and the actions that must be taken in order to meet them (Step 3).

Before we discuss approaches that I would not recommend, it is helpful to review five key points at which these methods fall short at providing long lasting solutions to emotional discomfort and distress. These points will also help you assess which models are helpful to you and which are not.

KNOW THE MISSING LINK

I have found that there are five reasons why other methods of emotional regulation may not work. These five reasons are in direct opposition with the five essential elements that are needed in order to make the processing of emotions functional and productive. And so when one or more of these key pieces are missing, they become the missing links that make those methods ineffective. So let's explore what they are.

Looking at the function of emotion — to signal as to whether or not our needs are met — it follows that in order to respond to an emotion properly we need two basic things. One is to understand that emotions reflect a particular need, and two — finding proper resources to meet those needs. To meet our needs appropriately, and thus respond to emotional signals in a functional way, we must complete a proper path from initially registering the signal to then finding resources to meet the need. This path consists of five essential elements, or links, which are:

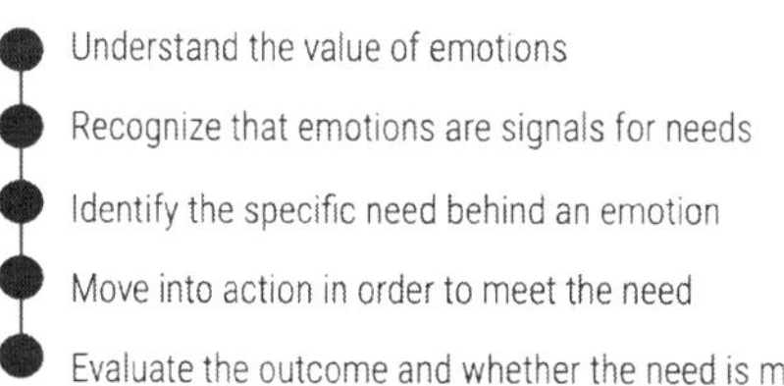

In order to receive the emotional signal to begin with, we have to want to receive it. Our ability to pay attention depends on our appreciation of emotions and whether we see them as signals worth paying attention to. But there is more. We also have to understand that an emotion is signaling to us about a need, and then proceed to figure out which need that is. And so on, down the path all the way through to the final element, which is — making sure our needs are actually met by the actions we took (i.e., resource/need match).

Each of the links in this process also serves as a point of potential failure in responding to emotions. In other words, when one or more of the essential links are omitted, it can lead to a dysfunctional response. A dysfunctional response is the kind of approach that fails to recognize and address the signal (i.e., the emotion and the need behind it). On the other hand, a functional response is the kind of action we take that helps us meet our needs.

Here is what the corresponding missing links look like when it comes to processing emotions incorrectly:

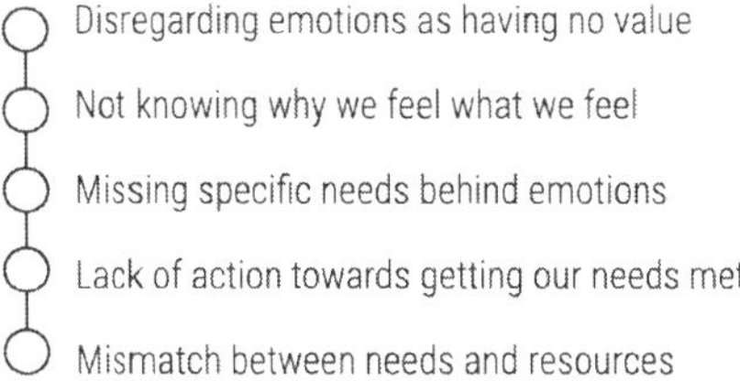

Notice that along this progression, there is absence of a desired outcome of resolving an emotion, which is — getting a need met. And that failure can happen at the very first point by dismissing emotions altogether or even at the last point, where the actions taken did not actually meet the need (even if there was an awareness of what that need was). The outcome of either of these points is an unmet need. That outcome will prompt the negative emotion to come up again and again, in higher intensity each time (remember the Unmet Need Arc we discussed earlier?). Not only that, but if we continue to dismiss the initial emotion, it is likely to get more confusing over time and get entangled with other feelings.

The good news is that each of these missing links has a corresponding appropriate action, which can help turn things around towards a functional outcome (i.e., meeting our needs). The table below gives you the dos and don'ts side by side for each of the essential links:

Essential Elements (DOs) ●-●-●-●-●	**Points of Failure (DON'Ts)** ○-○-○-○-○
✔ Understand the value of emotions	✘ Disregarding emotions as having no value
✔ Recognize that emotions are signals for needs	✘ Not knowing why we feel what we feel
✔ Identify the specific need behind an emotion	✘ Missing specific needs behind emotions
✔ Move into action in order to meet the need	✘ Lack of action towards getting our needs met
✔ Evaluate the outcome (whether the need is met)	✘ Mismatch between needs and resources

Keep this table in mind when you consider whether a particular model you are exploring for processing emotions is actually helpful. You see, most traditional and widely accepted models, especially the ones based in cognitive-behavioral therapy (CBT for short), stop us from exploring our needs. Many models guide us not to think about our emotions deeply altogether, which prevents us from understanding what we need and how to get it. Instead, we are directed to *change* our emotions. And we are told that the way to do it is by changing our thoughts.

This process is often referred to as "thought work," which means working on your thoughts to replace them with the ones that make you feel better. But that's where the misconception is. This is what stops us half-way from getting to where we need to go. You see, it isn't the thought that makes us feel better, it is the promise of a fulfilled need that does that. Believing that simply thinking different thoughts is enough, leads to a dysfunctional outcome of essentially distracting ourselves with other thoughts. Trying hard to convince ourselves that we feel something else, while ignoring what truly bothers us, is not going to make us feel better.

Instead of denying who we are, what we feel, and what matters to us, we must actually focus on fulfilling those needs and become more of who we are meant to be. A method that does not address underlying needs, cannot get us there.

We will *always* feel like something is missing or that the results we are getting don't last long enough. Regulating emotions without meeting our needs will *always* lead to the same outcomes, which is — unmet needs. And unmet needs, in turn, will *always* create ongoing negative experience and lingering dissatisfaction. So it makes me wonder, do these methods actually help resolve an emotion or do they create *an illusion* of that? That is for you to decide.

To help you navigate various methods out there and to better understand why I do not recommend certain approaches, I have added a link graphic to each category we will be discussing. Since each of the links is important, this visual will help you see how soon a particular approach fails at addressing the underlying reason behind the discomfort. As I review each approach, I will share my thoughts as to why a particular method breaks down at the point that it does. Here is a general overview of what the missing links represent:

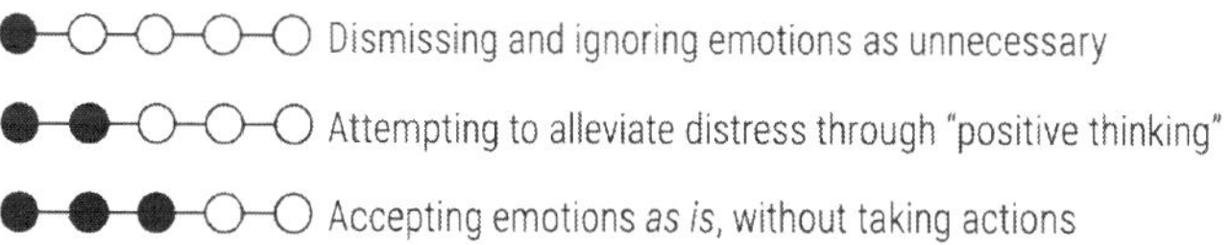

You will see that some models are missing several essentials, while others — just a couple. However, because *all five links are important*, the approaches included in this chapter do not really work (since they do not speak to the needs, let alone how to meet them). That is the reason why I do not recommend them, despite their widespread popularity.

Probably one of the reasons you are reading this book is because you've tried some of those popular methods and they haven't quite worked. Perhaps you've wondered why they were ineffective, so let's take a closer look to see what exactly they were missing.

SUPPRESSION & DENIAL

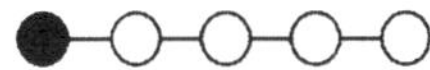

This category of recommendations for emotional regulation is what I call the "ignore yourself" camp. There are several strategies that fall into this school of thought. The basic premise of this approach is that emotions do not have value, that it is something that might have served us in the past, but is no longer necessary. We are told that emotions are not needed in modern life, as it is something that is rising from the older parts of the brain. That part of the brain, we are told, is called "the lizard brain" and that we need to evolve beyond that.

I must tell you that references to the lizard brain, also known as "reptilian brain," are misguided. At best, they are nothing more than a giant oversimplification of the brain, how it functions, and its evolutionary trajectory.

These references are based on a Triune Brain theory, an outdated hypothesis made in the 1960's by physician and neuroscientist Paul MacLean. Some people are relieved to hear that the reason why their behavior and emotions are so confusing and erratic is because there is an internal fight going on between not one, not two, but three (!) brains. Per this theory, the three different parts of the brain have their own, different, and often conflicting agendas. It's like a dinosaur, a monkey, and a computer put to work together — no wonder why humans do odd things! This would be a funny joke, except that many models of processing emotions were based on this incorrect assumption.

Although the theory has been since disproven as *conflicting with reality* by several studies, the myth of the lizard brain took hold in the vernacular of the self-help industry and pop-psychology. Despite multiple corrections published in the scientific literature since then, in attempts to stop this misconception from circulating, it is hard to terminate what appears to be a story too good not to repeat, and so it continues to spread even today.

If you have believed the story of the Triune Brain, let's course-correct going forward. Let this also be a lesson in the fallibility of the brightest of minds, and the fact that even the best theories and proposals have to be tested before they can be treated as facts. Let's also remember that even the biggest experts in the field make mistakes, which end up living a life of their own.

And while we're at it, let's also note that a hypothesis is just that — a hypothesis. Not only was this one not supported, but evidence to the contrary — disproving its accuracy — has been made available a long time ago. You may still hear people talk about "reptilian structures" in the brain, which suggests that they have not kept up with scientific retractions or may not be sensitive to the difference between hypotheses and hard facts. Perhaps you could share this book with them. Not only will it help correct said misconception, but also teach them a thing or two about what emotions are actually for and what to do about them.

Based on this widespread myth, people are told that "emotions make you weak" and so you have to "be bigger than your emotions" and "cut them out, like weeds." How do you do that? By training your mind, you are being instructed. By getting "tougher." By using logic and by training your will. You are supposed to will your way over fear, will over anger, and will over sadness. The mind is seen as the master, as the domineering part, the one that has to gain control over emotions. If it doesn't, then one becomes a victim to their feelings.

What do you hear in these words? I hear struggle, a fight, and an internal battle of thoughts over feelings, words over sensations.

And since, clearly, emotions within this category of methods are seen as something negative, there is a lot of shame associated with feeling them. Whenever we invite shame into our life, the natural reaction will be to deny or suppress whatever makes us feel it.

All of this leads to intentional rejection of emotions. And, since emotions are so core to who we are and what we need, rejecting them also means rejecting yourself. Some people get so good at suppressing their feelings, they altogether fail to notice they have them, let alone be able to tell what it is that they are actually feeling. And if this is where we are at, then we are far from finding resources for our needs. There is no space for them in this conversation, just like there is no space for emotions.

As you can see, when evaluated against our five essential elements, this type of approach most definitely breaks down at the very first point, which is "missing the signal." In fact, proponents of this approach consider it an *accomplishment* to not feel negative emotions and, therefore, they miss the opportunity to truly get in touch with what is off.

When we do not understand what feelings are for, we think they are not useful.

Not only we think of them as not useful, we will also perceive them as getting in the way of us living our best life. So we think, if we could just learn to ignore our feelings, learn not to show them (even to ourselves), then we will be able to do the things we want to do in life. And yet, the opposite is actually true. The more we ignore how we feel, the less likely we are to take the right steps to get to what we want. As we have discussed throughout this book, it is our feelings that tell us what is missing, what is needed, and what may be a good resource to meet our needs.

I hope, when you come across these types of models and methods, you will discard them. They have very little to offer, because right out the gate they devalue the very thing that helps us make sense of our experience as human beings — our emotions.

GIMMICKS & WORD PLAY

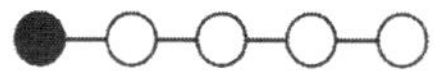

This one is, what I call, the "trick yourself" camp. Although it relies on a whole different set of tactics, it is just as bad as the previous type of methods that we discussed above. It uses turns of phrase and tricks of the tongue to downplay emotional sensations and to redirect attention to something else. It stems from a pseudo-scientific, yet well absorbed into the mainstream, approach known as neuro-linguistic programming (NLP for short). These approaches rely on language to "program" your mind so that you *see* things differently from how you *actually experience* them.

There is no empirical, practical, hands-on support for these methods. In other words, in order for this to work you must *believe* it works. So it isn't the process or the method that makes regulating emotions effective, but how much you *believe* what you are telling yourself about it. At best, this is the placebo effect at play if you believe in the "magic of words." But what is more concerning is that it is a form of denial of your own *direct experience*, since its purpose is to redirect you from your experience and your emotions.

Cute or catchy, this type of method looks at words as means of distracting you from your actual experience. And it may include such linguistic devices as rhyming, alliteration, clever acronyms, repetition, oxymorons, paradoxes, etc. Without these linguistic devices, the "magic" of these methods falls apart.

So when it comes to processing emotions, you may hear things like: "Turn that frown upside down." That means to change your perspective (as in flipping the curve of the sad mouth upside down to turn it into a smiley one). A change of perspective may be a great thing. But when it comes to emotions, this is not a helpful suggestion. In other words, you are advised to feel better by simply changing your perspective, as in, telling yourself you are just looking at things backwards. This often includes dismissing the reality of what you are experiencing.

Don't like a frown? No worries! Turn it upside down and it will look like a smile. *Look like...* That is all we are likely to accomplish using gimmicks like that, and that is — *an appearance* of change. We both know that an emotional experience has nothing to do with lines on paper or pictographs, like emojis.

Of course there is no denying the power of words.

Still, do we want to believe in "word magic"?

The only thing that works like magic is when we get our needs met.

It is important you learn to see these tricks for what they are. Language, of course, is a powerful tool and often the one we ignore. So yes, paying attention to what we are saying can change how we think about things. However, when it comes to emotions, we wouldn't want to be changing our words in order to not feel emotions. That's the wrong approach and goes against everything we talked about in this book.

Of course it is helpful to see if how we speak limits our abilities and resources. Certain phrases can keep us stuck. Recognizing this is especially useful when we are trying to figure out how to meet our needs and what resources to go after. On the flip side, however, language manipulation can be just as unhelpful by presenting you with new linguistic traps to replace the old ones. And that is exactly what happens when we trick ourselves out of feelings by using certain catch-phrases, as in these examples:

✘ "*E*-motion is *Energy* in Motion"

✘ "Fear is *F.E.A.R.*" (*F*alse *E*vidence *A*ppearing *R*eal)

You may have seen these and other similar memes about emotions. These are examples of linguistic trickery. I call it trickery because not only does it fail to reflect the truth of what is real, but it is often used *to mask* the reality of our experience.

But how can we tell that this language does not represent reality? One simple way is to realize that these phrases do not survive translation and do not work in other languages. If the concept is held together with carefully selected words and words alone, then there is no real meaning behind it. For example, the word "emotion" in other languages does not have the same components that could stand for "energy" and "motion." This makes the phrase "*E*-motion is *Energy* in Motion" highly dubious. Same goes for fear. In other languages, the spelling of the word "fear" cannot be used to make the same acronym to communicate the same message in regards to "false evidence."

Therefore, these phrases do not serve as confirmations for what is real and true, but rather they illustrate the purely coincidental nature of word play. Real truth cannot be dependent on the stability and strength of linguistic constructs. Some may argue (and that is the whole premise of neuro-linguistic programming) that language "constructs reality," and I certainly think that it does create *filters* through which we *view reality*.

However, the emphasis I am placing here is not on the *power* of language but rather on its *limitations*, especially when it comes to articulating the reality of our emotional experience. Furthermore, the second point I am making is that we can tell without a doubt when the words we use fail to represent reality. And that is, when their inability to carry the same meaning across the globe, across cultures, and across translations, is so — obvious.

On the other hand, something that is naturally true, will preserve its essence and its meaning, no matter who speaks of it and in what language. If the meaning gets lost when the words change or their spelling is different, we have an issue of a linguistic illusion. Only those things are true about emotions that remain to be true no matter which culture we think of or what language is used to speak about them, *if at all*. Here I am reminding you of the conversation we had in Chapter 2, where we specifically talked about the *pre-verbal* quality of emotions. The pre-verbal nature of emotions means that language has little to do with the reality and the essence of our basic emotional experiences.

Therefore, using linguistic tricks to dismiss emotions does not really work. Not to mention, the mere fact that such linguistic constructs collapse when translated into another language, says everything we need to know about their validity, their ability to communicate what is real, and, consequently, how seriously they should be taken.

And when it comes to the phrase related to fear in particular (i.e., "fear is *f*-alse *e*-vidence *a*-ppearing *r*-eal"), regardless of what you know about its linguistic vulnerabilities, I have a hunch that you wouldn't like hearing someone tell you that your fear is imagined. How does that phrase make you feel? Dismissed and invalidated, I'm sure. This is the biggest example of reality-denial I've seen so far. What this teaches us to do is to look at our experience of fear and simply deny it, since the first word that comes out of our mouth when we say the phrase "false evidence appearing real" is *"false."* And just like that, right out the gate, we are told to dismiss the reality of what we are feeling and why.

But let's slow down for a minute... Who says fear *is* false? And who says we need *actual* evidence of danger in order to worry? Quite the opposite. If we understand the function of emotion to signal to us about our needs, we can see that fear is serving the same function — telling us about our needs, current and future ones. Fear has a *protective* factor, so that we are ready "just in case" and so a lot of that will depend on our ability to foresee danger *before* we have evidence for it. I could go on and on about the purpose of emotions, but let's return to linguistic tricks and what to be aware of.

The more catchy are the phrases, the more likely they are to be repeated. That's how they spread.

However, repeating something doesn't make it true.

So whenever you hear some clever wording about emotions, ask yourself: "It *sounds* clever... but does it *feel* true?" Ask yourself if what you are hearing is simply the trick of language and if so, don't adopt it. It is an *illusion* of truth rather than a representation of truth. Pretentious "truths," that are only "true" in the language they are spoken in, do not express universal or natural truths. They may express cultural beliefs but do not have universal application. And, as we know, when it comes to emotions, given how core they are to any human being across cultures and languages, the truth about our experience of them must not be limited to the language used to describe them. So if words and phrases you hear about emotions have limitations to how true they are, then they are not so true after all, are they?

They are simply tricks, intentional ways to trick the mind.

And, if you think of it, that actually makes sense for the proponents of this particular school of thought, where the objective is, in fact, to trick the mind about emotions. That's the whole point, the trickery is what these models openly pride themselves on. If you think about it, the way they look at the brain when it comes to emotions is that they perceive the brain as "playing tricks" on us (e.g., warning us of the dangers that supposedly aren't there, and so on). And so, from that perspective, it is only fair to trick it back or get back at it with clever (or so they think) word play.

But what happens in reality is that tricks like that distract you. They only provide a temporary relief, like all distractions do. However, what we truly need are real answers and resolution.

This category, therefore, also has too many missing links. It fails to address your needs as early as the first point of failure, because it attempts to distract you from emotions. Although it does acknowledge their existence, it gives them no value, and does not help you understand what you are feeling or why. It is unhelpful to believe you are making changes in your life (by turning that frown upside down), when in fact you continue to be stuck.

Whereas the previous category of methods come across as somewhat severe and oppressive in their resolve to "fight" against emotions, this one comes across as rather playful. However, that playfulness in this context makes it immature and dismissive of emotions. Though this school of thought may not see emotions as "the enemy," it does look at them as something trivial and to be treated with frivolity. That is why I recommend skipping these methods. They will not teach you to take care of your needs.

POSITIVE AFFIRMATIONS

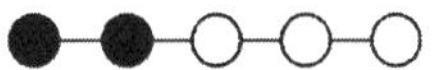

Have you noticed that it is the people that do not have solutions for you who will often tell you that the answer to your problems is your mindset? And that in order to feel positive, you need to use positive statements and affirmations. I am not saying mindset is not important. Mindset is a form of attitude, a perspective we take on things, and so of course it is important. However, when it comes to finding answers to our challenges, having a great attitude alone is not going to be enough. It is like a great sauce to a dish, but not the dish itself. What *does* resolve our challenges is looking at what is *needed* and what *resources* are available to address that particular need.

According to recommendations that belong to this category of methods, when we feel negative emotions we need to regulate them with positive self-affirming statements. We are told to repeat these statements several times, for as long as needed, until we feel positive emotions. Here is what these affirmations may sound like:

"My life is stress-free"

"I let go of fear, I let go of anger"

"I choose how I want to feel"

"I have power over my emotions"

"I am at peace with everything"

So when an unpleasant emotion shows up, these statements are intended to shift our attention to positive things. Although positive statements have their value, making these types of statements at a time of struggle may feel almost out-of-touch with reality. Moreover, although generally speaking positive statements can be self-affirming and reassuring, when they are out of alignment with the situation itself — they do not feel validating. Why is that?

If you recall our conversation about validation and acknowledgement in Chapter 7, you may remember that the true power of acknowledgment and validation lies in its *profound* ability to speak to *the truth of one's experience*. In other words, real acknowledgement and validation feel deeply reaffirming because they speak to what is true for us and our present experience, whereas positive affirmations offer statements that feel far from *the truth of the moment*. That is the reason why they do not feel validating. And that is also the reason why they don't work well.

In order to force them to work, people are instructed to repeat an affirmation of choice many times. This is not surprising because saying something we do not believe only once has no impact, but repeating something *as many times as needed* does accomplish the goal of inserting that thought into our mind.

Once that insertion happens, it initiates its own cycle of repetition, like an earworm (something you might have experienced if you ever had a song or a tune stuck in your head). Of course, one might argue that if you are to have earworms, it is better if they sound like positive affirmations. That sounds like settling for less, and we deserve better than that. I would rather have no earworms at all by being intentional and aware about what I am thinking. Not to mention that, if our goal is to resolve emotional discomfort, affirmations do little to address the core of this issue.

The reason this strategy has some effect is because it has the ability to induce a hypnotic state, thus making the mind susceptible to *believing* something that may not be reflective of our reality. That is why I think of this category of recommendations as the "self-hypnosis" camp. Affirmations and mantras in their repetitive nature are supposed to influence our subconscious. However, the challenge we run into with this, is that in order to understand your emotions and which needs they communicate about, we have to engage actively and consciously. We have to have full awareness and be in the presence of what is going on for us. Only this way will we be able to understand what around us has shifted to contribute to how we may be feeling. The part that is most unhelpful about this type of approach is the redirection of our attention away from the very thing what we actually must pay attention to (i.e., our emotions and needs).

There is danger of positive thinking of this kind.

When disconnected from reality, it leads to negative results and dysfunctional outcomes. Think about it... How often do people resort to positive affirmations to convince themselves of looking the other way, to ignore what is true, to disconnect from pain? Very often, because that is exactly what affirmations are for. And how many of these people have genuinely solved their concerns through affirmations? Not many. Affirmations make you too numb and disconnected to understand what you were feeling and why. Plus the false sense of wellbeing (i.e., superficially induced "positive mindset") prevents you from acknowledging that something is not working to begin with. Why would I be attempting to solve anything if *"My life is stress-free" "I let go of fear" "I let go of anger" and "I am at peace with everything"*? Exactly.

Truly positive outcomes come from thinking which is grounded in reality. That reality is the reality of what we perceive, experience, feel, think, and need.

Only after taking it all in for internal assessment can we make the best choice of how to move forward towards a better outcome. The only positive thinking that can be positive for us is the kind of thinking that results in taking actions towards the outcomes we want. This is the exact opposite of the type of thinking that keeps our eyes closed, makes us stay still, waiting until the unpleasant reality walks away on its own. This kind of thinking, which does not move us into action, is going to have negative outcomes.

It is similar to what one does on a walk where, instead of paying attention to a sprained ankle and making sure they walk carefully so as to not injure themselves any further, they are being encouraged to look at the flowers and enjoy the fresh air. And are being advised to say things like: "I am here to enjoy nature. I am not here to worry about my ankle." But how is this helpful? What's wrong with the *both/and* approach? Why can't we enjoy nature, while *also* making sure we are paying attention to the sprained ankle? If you don't pay attention *to both*, you're more likely to end up with more pain and exacerbate the injury.

Attending to our needs does not mean we disregard what's wonderful. Likewise, we cannot use what's wonderful against ourselves to disregard what isn't so wonderful.

Engaging in "positive thinking" while experiencing negative emotions will result in denial of our true experience. It will make us ignore not only our emotional signals and the messages behind them (i.e., unmet needs), but also what made us feel that way in the first place (i.e., changes in our surroundings). Positive thinking results in neglect of our needs, which in the end is going to bring more suffering. If we have a hunch that our negative reality arises only from our thinking style and our mindset, then yes, we can try to think positively as a way of finding better actions and choices that can help change that reality into a more positive one.

But this is wrong when it comes to our needs, because our needs do not arise from "negative thinking" and, because of that, they are not solved with "positive thinking." A negative experience, which is experienced as such through our emotions (and not thoughts), is a sign of unmet needs. These needs have to be met, and that is where the action comes in.

When we act to meet the need (the presence of which is signaled through an emotion), *we change* our experience into a more positive one.

This works so much better than the self-induced hypnosis, which does not remove the pain — only *your awareness* of it.

However, if we want to resolve challenges, we need *more* awareness, not less. So my strong recommendation is to stay grounded in the reality of what you feel and to become aware of your needs. And let that guide your thinking and your actions. When we deny what we feel, by trying to replace our thoughts in hopes of replacing our feelings, what ends up happening is a huge invalidation of ourselves. We end up lying to ourselves and forcing ourselves to accept our own lies. This leads to high-tension internal conflict, which we attempt to resolve by doing more of the same — trying to change how we think about it. It doesn't work.

Of course, our beliefs can get in the way of us getting what we want, in which cases we do need new and better beliefs. However, in order for a new belief to have the power to change things for the better, it has to drive the right action that will help us achieve what we are after.

Changes in life happen when we are actively engaged with life.

Affirmations alone cannot do that.

They plant statements in our mind that suggest that our reality is already the way we want it to be. If that is truly so, then there are no actions we need to take to change anything. However, if that is not so, then saying affirmations ultimately does not help us meet our needs that prompted the emotional discomfort in the first place.

In order to have an impact on our reality, we have to have an intent.

We must act, not just think.

Like I said earlier, mindset is the sauce, not the dish itself. And for all these reasons, this category of methods has several missing links and breaks down at the second essential element. Although this type of approach is definitely better than the two we explored previously (since it does not engage in internal battles or trickery of the brain), it is still rather ineffective.

It gets us a little bit further along, because it does acknowledge the presence of emotion and it does not actively make emotions be a bad thing. However, since it has nothing else to offer, it invites you to distract yourself from emotions and, in doing so, dismisses them. So, although something like this may provide short-term relief, it is not addressing the core reason behind our emotions. And even though it does register the signal, it is misunderstanding what the signal is for. Therefore, it is offering ineffective recommendations on how to process emotions.

CHANGING YOUR THOUGHTS

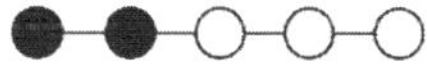

Here we are talking about any modalities and tactics that focus on identifying thoughts as the cause of emotions and that perceive "working on thoughts" as the answer to emotional discomfort. In this category, there are several different models with different names, but all of them are based on the principles of cognitive-behavioral therapy (CBT for short), which originated in the 1960's.

This category of models and approaches is also missing several critical links and most of them break down at the second essential element (i.e., recognizing that emotions are signals for needs). In many ways, these approaches are similar to the affirmations in terms of what they accomplish. Or rather, what they fail to accomplish (i.e., finding a need and addressing it). However, they go about it in a different and more involved way, and that is why this category deserves its own separate section. Whereas the affirmations-based method invites you to just think of something else and be positive, the change-your-thoughts methods are actively engaging you in the process of changing your emotions through *thinking* about them in a very specific prescriptive way.

I call these methods, especially the way they have evolved in the mainstream self-help culture, the "brainwash yourself" camp. Why? Because these techniques resemble forceful methods of thought control and coercive self-persuasion. The only difference from the actual brainwashing is that we are invited to do this *voluntarily to ourselves*, rinse-and-repeat style, all the time and any time, whenever an emotion we do not like arises.

Now, it must be said that these methods were not designed to be coercive or harmful. Nor were they intended to lead to self-directed brainwashing.

Similar to the "lizard brain" hypothesis, these were some models proposed in the earlier days *to help* us process emotions and *help us* regulate emotional experiences. And in some limited ways they do succeed. They offer a change in perspective that allows us to gain *temporary relief* from our situation and our painful feelings.

However, because they are either completely incorrect (as is the case with the "lizard brain" myth) or are incomplete (as cognitive-behavioral approaches tend to be), they do not address what is asking to be addressed, which is — our needs. In fact, our needs never play a role in any of these models, because of the basic premise they are built on that puts *thoughts*, not *unmet needs*, at the core of all painful experiences.

The basic premise of the various models within this approach is that thoughts cause emotions.

And so the proposed solution is to "work on your thoughts."

We are constantly (but erroneously) told that no one and nothing in our environment can cause us to feel anything. Another way of saying this is that circumstances (e.g., people, places, and things) are neutral, and that it's our thoughts that give it context and make it be a negative or a positive experience. We are told that it is our thoughts that create the feeling in the context of the circumstance. They tell you that in order to feel better you have to decide what feeling you want to feel and then choose a thought that would match that feeling. The whole game, you are told, starts and ends in your mind. These models also postulate that thoughts have a specific predetermined charge — positive or negative (as in, positive thoughts give you positive feelings and negative thoughts give you negative feelings) — but this isn't so.

This type of teaching openly challenges you to test this idea of "environmental neutrality" by arguing that two different people will have two different reactions to the same circumstance, to the same event. Therefore, they say, this is evidence that events in our lives and circumstances in our environment are neutral, and that we are the ones that turn them into problems because of the way we think about them. If only we were willing to change our thinking and manage our mind, they say, then we would have positive emotions, generated by positive thinking. This is nonsense and we will get to that in a minute.

The circumstances of our experience can never be neutral.

Why is that?

Because it is *our* experience.

Our experience will be a positive one if it is meeting our needs and a negative one if it doesn't. And our emotions reflect exactly that. What we feel tells us whether our experience is in alignment with our needs or not. And so our experience is *meant to be subjective.* So then, with this in mind, the neutrality argument does not even apply here, whatsoever. It is not relevant. For example, what does it matter if other people are not cold — I am. Whether other people are bothered by wind or not does not prevent *me* from taking care of *me*. What does it matter if other people do not like rain, I do. And so *I* am going to enjoy it. We're all unique individuals. That's the beauty, not a problem.

When we focus on the thoughts in order to change how we feel, we are trying to convince our mind that the reality of our experience is not what it is and that it is supposed to be "neutral." But no, it isn't *supposed* to be neutral. It is supposed to be *subjective*, based on who we are and our unique needs.

Let's also look at the fact that not only do people have different reactions to events, they also have different emotional reactions to the *thoughts* themselves. To me this indicates that a thought itself is not guaranteed to produce a positive feeling. A positively-phrased thought may produce a negative feeling, just as a negatively-phrased thought may produce a positive feeling. It all depends on how appropriate the initial thought is for the situation. Not only that, but also how *aligned* that thought is with what is actually happening.

Notice too, how internally we have a natural resistance — a reaction of rejection — to a thought that may be positively phrased but is not aligned with what we truly feel. For example, someone made a rude comment to you and your friend says: "C'mon, get over it! He didn't really mean it. It would be more helpful to think that he meant it as a compliment!" Those are *positive* thoughts we would have *negative* thoughts about, and will feel compelled to reject.

Spontaneous thoughts *reflect* how we feel. This can only happen because spontaneous thoughts are formed from our feelings, not the other way around. And so, what is *actually* happening can only be understood through the frame of our *own* reference, through the frame of our *own* meaning-making, and our *own* needs.

In other words, what is happening is *never* neutral.

Meaning, it is never neutral if it *matters* to us.

And if it happens to be neutral, then it is not relevant to us and not meaningful enough. Therefore, it does not apply to us and we move on. Before we jump on the bandwagon of changing our thoughts and changing our interpretation — and therefore changing the meaning — we should first ask: *Why* am I reacting to such-and-such? What about this is *meaningful* to me? What does this meaning tell me about *my needs and values*? Knowing our values and needs helps us understand what, if anything, can be done about this particular situation or experience. "Working on our thoughts" is the last thing we should be doing in an effort to meet our needs. Forced positive thoughts do not reflect how we feel. They attempt to induce a feeling that is not there.

Since I just mentioned "interpretation" and since this is something these methods try to tackle as a way of regulating emotion, let me say a couple of things about it. Proponents of the CBT-type models tell you that interpretations themselves are the problem. In fact, they tell you, that this is why we live miserable lives — because we interpret things. We use our thoughts in the wrong way, they say. We should try our best to not have any interpretations. That is what will allow us to see the worlds and events around us as neutral.

But in reality — we do interpret.

And that is not a curse. It's a blessing.

That is what makes us uniquely human, as well as *uniquely us* amongst other humans. To be able to receive and interpret various signals is actually a special capacity that we have developed over the years. And the reason why we interpret things is because we are meaning-making beings.

That's a good thing! That is why we are able to evolve as humans, because we are able to make meaning, understand our experiences, and grow from them. So what these models do is they tell you that making meaning somehow is a problem, which consequently conveys the idea that we absolutely must change the way we make meaning of things in order to feel better.

But the problem is — that does not work.

Why?

Because it is important to interpret.

Not only that, but it is important to interpret things with our own mind, from our own perspective, and through the filter of our own needs. It is important to make meaning based on our needs. The only difference is that — when we do interpret — we must learn to interpret events and circumstances accurately. Meaning, as a reflection of our needs, what works for us, and what doesn't. It is vital that we do that as humans in order to keep our needs in balance, to keep growing and evolving. The goal is not to try and make everything into a positive, but to interpret accurately, which means we have to know ourselves and our needs.

- Our values, as well as our needs, dictate how we will make meaning about what is happening to us.

That is not a bad thing. That is actually a good thing. In order to live full, complete, and meaningful lives, we must live in accordance with our values, while at the same time be able to meet our needs along the way.

If we stop interpreting life events, we will stop making sense out of what is happening to us, with us, and around us. This will lead to a life devoid of meaning. Now, let me ask you, how excited are you to live a life without meaning?

- Loss of meaning leads to loss of vitality.

So the key here is not to stop interpreting circumstances and life events, but rather to be aware of what influences our ability to interpret them accurately. And let's be mindful of whether our interpretations are in alignment with our needs and our values.

But how do we explain that different people have different emotional reactions to the same circumstance? Simple. It is because the same situation may be meeting the needs of some people and not meeting the needs of others.

For example, when two teams face off in a tournament, one team's win will cause joy to one person while at the same time cause disappointment to another. And this isn't happening because one person has the "right thoughts" and another one has the "wrong thoughts," but because a loss is just as meaningful as a win when it is *your team*.

So yes, we have a different reaction to a situation because we have a different interpretation of it. True. But is it proper to say that we have the "wrong" reaction or that we have the "wrong" interpretation? Not at all!

We will always have our own unique interpretation, because it comes from who we are, what we need, where we find meaning, and what we value. Our interpretations are not wrong when they align with what is happening for us. Nothing is wrong with mourning a loss, even if the same event is the cause for celebration for someone else. It would be completely backwards to try and celebrate a loss, no? Sounds like nonsense, because it is.

Believing our own nonsense is the most dangerous thing.

It leads us down the path of self-deception.

Let's not fall for our own gibberish and try to convince ourselves that our thoughts know better. CBT-based models, similar to affirmations, is a form of self-denial that can lead to incongruent feelings, a contradiction between our emotional experience and our forced positive thoughts about it. Brainwashing yourself into believing things you don't actually believe is the worst form of self deception.

This type of practice also makes you susceptible to other people's brainwashing. If you accept your own lies, you will accept them from others too. Just like you would use discernment and vet what others tell you, you should do the same with the thoughts and messages you are asked to *force* upon yourself. Anything done with force and against our gut sense, is inherently wrong.

So how do we resolve this conundrum?

The only way is to look at the missing pieces which are our values and our needs. These dictate whether something is perceived to be in alignment (i.e., positive signal) or not (i.e., negative signal).

This is the reason why "thoughtwork" can so often feel out of alignment with ourselves and can create so much resistance around it, because it rarely resonates with *what feels true*. We will naturally feel resistance to placing other people's thoughts and feelings into our mind. That is why we feel resistance when we are asked to change how we experience reality and how we interpret our experience. This kind of resistance is actually a very healthy response to thoughtwork and to CBT-based models. Why? Because it is a healthy way of rejecting invalidation and subversion.

This response is a reflection of a natural boundary we put around ourselves and our experience. This is how we protect what matters.

Whenever you are confused, it is always helpful to fall back on what *you* know to be true. How do you know something rings true? Because of how you *feel*. And no, you don't feel a particular way because of your thinking. We don't try to change how we feel if what we feel is true, which — it always is.

The only reason why we try to change how we think is because models of this kind make us believe that our feelings are not the truth. But it is. It is our own Truth. It is the *truth of our experience* (which is always reflective of who we are, our values and needs).

- We can only live our lives in accordance with *our* Truth, *our* Values, and *our* Needs.

As kind, respectful, and compassionate humans, we do not invalidate other people's values, we do not reject their needs as unreal, and we do not reject or try to change their feelings. So why then do we do this to ourselves? Because models like these make us believe that this is a shortcut to happiness. It never is.

The more incongruent our thoughts are with what we feel, the more disconnected we are from ourselves. Internal disconnect is never the way to happiness. I do not recommend it.

WATCHING YOUR EMOTIONS

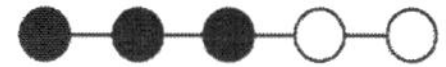

If it sounds like you are about to watch a movie, you are on the right track. This is sort of what this school of thought is inviting you to do. To watch your emotions from aside, to observe them come and go. Observe yourself having an experience, as if someone else's, as if in a movie. That is all. Oh, and have fun, if you can manage.

The premise is that by watching your emotions, like a movie that plays out in front of you, you eventually feel better. Since you are not getting too involved in them personally, you detach yourself from what is happening. That detachment, according to this approach, is considered to be the answer to emotional regulation.

This is what I call the "sit with it" camp. You are invited to "sit with your emotion" as opposed to change them or manipulate your mind out of them. And this is what I appreciate the most about this school of thought. Not only are they accepting and welcoming of all emotions, they see them as valid and worth having.

This practice and view of emotions is in alignment with Step One of the 3-Step Needs-Based Process we have discussed in this book. And so this approach is by far the best amongst other methods out there.

However, this is also the only thing I like about it. These approaches are still quite incomplete in meeting our needs when used on their own. Even though they get us even further along than any other methods we have discussed so far, they still have two critical missing links to resolving emotions fully. One such key element is developing awareness of the *needs* behind the emotion and the other — finding *resources* to meet them.

Whereas the other methods lean heavily into The Mind and instruct us to push through our emotions with the power of will and thinking, this school of thought invites you to connect with The Body instead. I deeply appreciate the notion of sensing our emotion as a whole-body experience, because it is, naturally so. It is a sensation that arises within our body. Emotions show up *in the body* for a reason, because they are meant to engage the body into action once our needs become clear.

By design, emotions apply to our *whole being* and our ability to *keep being*, to keep living, our sense of aliveness, to our survival. Because of that, our body does have to be engaged in order to resolve negative emotions.

Even though we use our mind when we get in touch with the need and try to figure out what resources to reach for, we still have to engage our body to get those needs met. In fact, we can never "solve it" with our brain alone and think our way out of emotions (which is something CBT-based models teach you to do). We need to truly feel our feelings — in our whole body — in order to fully understand what is going on for us. And once that is clear, we can move into action to meet our needs.

Another reason why these methods get us further along than other tricks and strategies, is that there is no judging of emotions, and you are not asked to do any "thoughtwork." You are not even asked to try to change what you are feeling. You are just seeing what is, allowing it to show up, express itself, and then let it go.

The language around all of these directions is peaceful and welcoming, as you may have sensed yourself. However, oftentimes it is not clear what it actually means to "sit with it" or to "watch it" and many people find this process a bit frustrating and vague.

This is where methods in this category fall short. And that is understandable. The lack of clarity when it comes to directions of how to "be with your emotions" is rooted in a lack of comprehension of the actual purpose behind our emotions. And without the awareness of the role emotions play, the process of "sitting with it" may actually lead to overwhelm. Being in full presence of emotions that feel overpowering and do nothing about them, can make some people feel lost in that emotion, overtaken by it.

It's all well and good when emotions are perceived as a form of energy, that ebbs and flows, and is seen as something natural. The problem, however, is when this energy is perceived as "out there," flowing in and out, coming and going, as if unrelated to us. No wonder why, from that perspective, we are told that it is useless to do anything about it, that we should not even try to interpret the energy of emotions or get involved in it. The proponents of this method often speak of emotions as "energy in motion" (which we discussed earlier), and this is exactly the part that I find unhelpful.

The sit-with-it guidance is not specific enough to understand what to do, besides sitting there and watching emotions come and go. How do you "watch to your emotions"? How long is enough? What do you do after that? What if the feeling is not going away? It is unclear. You are not offered much guidance around these questions. Instead, you are instructed to tune into the perceived attributes of an emotion, such as color, location, and shape.

This is problematic, and here is why.

By telling all these "stories" about the emotion, we misdirect our attention and overuse our mind to describe the feeling, as opposed to understanding what it is about. And the irony is that what started out as an *em-bodied experience*, now turns into a brainy process. As opposed to the whole-body inner knowing of what one feels (and, consequently, what one needs), we insert the mind by asking the wrong questions: "Is it heavy, or it is light?" "Does it flutter like a butterfly, or is it as hard as a rock?" "Is it blue and shimmery, or is it purple and pulsating?"

These descriptions of emotions are not that useful.

They distract us and do not lead us anywhere.

In my opinion, this is only worth paying attention to as a means of increasing your awareness of you feeling *something*. But if you spend too much time here, what you end up doing is actually distracting yourself from the emotion and the purpose behind it, even though it may seem like you *are* paying attention. I know, twisted, right?

Let me explain this part a bit more.

How is it that in describing color, size, and shape, we are not focusing on the emotion? You see, by assigning all these visual, tactile, and other sensorial attributes to emotions, we pay attention to the wrong things. In doing so, we stop asking: what the emotion is for, what is it there to tell us about our needs?

Understandably, this is not something these models teach, and so you wouldn't know to ask about it, if this is all you knew about emotions. But as we walked through the 3-Step Needs-Based Process in this book, you now know that this is one of the most important questions to be asking. This is how we get to understand what needs an emotion is signaling to us about.

- Gaining awareness of our needs
  does not depend on our ability to describe any of the sensorial aspects of an emotion.

These distractions may do the job of alleviating the feeling of discomfort, because your mind will be preoccupied with other aspects you tell yourself are important (such as the color and the shape of your sensation). This may distract you from the emotion, making it less intense in the moment, which temporarily may feel better. However, if this is all you settle for, it will not offer you any answers nor additional benefits of getting your needs met, which is ultimately what builds your inner strength and your capacity to embrace — and even benefit from — life's challenges.

Don't get me wrong. Of course, I am appreciating how much space is given to the actual acceptance of emotions and developing awareness of them. There is more allowing and acknowledging of emotions here, than there is in any other methods. It takes us out of our heads and into the body, which is incredibly important, since this is where emotions present themselves. This type of approach really helps you get comfortable feeling a whole range of experiences without rejecting them. At the same time, however, to truly resolve what an emotion brings up, we have to complete the full process by meeting the underlying need.

And that is where these methods, too, fall short.

It is the passivity of this approach when it comes to emotions that is particularly unhelpful. Not only is there no introspection to ask yourself why you feel the way you feel and to understand your inner workings better, but it is also missing the point that the only way to feel good is to have your needs met.

Sure, the emotion will finally fade away (following the Need Arc we discussed in Chapter 7), but what it was pointing to — the need itself — is not seen and, therefore, is not likely to be resolved.

When the emotion lessens in intensity and fades, we may get the impression that we truly resolved it. But how could we have? Resolved means — I understood what the need was, I took action, and I met the need. Resolved does not mean — I just forgot about it, moved on from it, or it is simply not bothering me anymore. As a result, this unmet need will prompt the emotion to come back and try to gain our attention. At which point your only option, per this method, is to "sit with it" yet again.

The 3-Step Needs-Based Process I have described in this book allows you not only to "sit-with-it" but also to understand what to *do-with-it*, by asking a series of questions. These questions were discussed in the earlier chapters and cover each of the three areas of awareness: emotions, needs, and resources.

Chapter 10

Values, Priorities, & Guilt

The focus of this book has been on emotional regulation. So far we've talked about how to process emotions, how to understand our needs, and how to seek appropriate resources to meet them. All three components of the 3-Step Needs-Based Process work together to ensure you know how you feel, why, and what to do about it. Throughout the book, we've touched upon a couple of concepts that would be helpful to give a little bit of additional air time in this final chapter.

One of them is *values.*

Another is — *priorities.*

And the third one is — *guilt.*

And these are not that separate from each other. Quite the opposite, they influence one another. Let me show you. Your values set your priorities and guide how you navigate situations when resources are limited. And when you do set your priorities, you may have a feeling of guilt rise up, especially if you are prioritizing something important to you as opposed to what others expect you to.

Not only do values guide us to discover what is truly important to us in our unique expression of needs, they also help set boundaries with other people, which in turn helps us manage guilt. A strong alignment with our values frees us from guilt because we end up acting with integrity and responsibility, in accordance with our values, standards, and morals. It may be surprising at first, but as you explore these areas with me, you will see that values play a critical role in our ability to meet our needs. Having strong clear values is a personal asset, and as such, you can consider them part of your arsenal of resources.

So let's chat about all that before you go.

WHAT DO VALUES HAVE TO DO WITH IT

Processing emotions properly requires taking action, and that is why taking action is an inseparable part of the 3-Step Needs-Based Process. What actions we take and how we decide to meet our needs largely depends on our values. Without taking action, we are unlikely to meet our needs, and without clear values our actions may be less intentional and lack confidence.

Not only do values help us make decisions (to make sure they align with the integrity of who we are), but they also have a way of reaffirming our worth and value, which is what gives us confidence. In addition to that, values help us live a life of purpose, which happens to be one of 8 Core Psychological Needs.

All of this is true when we *know* our values.

Not knowing your values, does not mean you don't have them.

We always have values, because it is something deeply integral to our nature as a human being. Our values allow us to bring our own perspective to the world. However, when we are not as clear about what our values are, we may have difficulty expressing them in our actions and don't use them to our advantage. Values, just like needs, change and evolve over time because we, too, evolve and change over time. Not only does it help to know your values, but it is also useful to revisit and review them every once in a while.

Although there are many lists of values available out there, for the sake of convenience I am offering you one in Appendix C of this book. It is, by no means, an exhaustive list and so, if some of your personal values are not on that list, please go ahead and write them in.

So what is the purpose of values? Values guide our decisions, actions, and choices, and they serve as an internal system of beliefs and attitudes that together work as our own internal compass. This is especially helpful when faced with life's challenges and when we find ourselves at crossroads trying to choose the right path. Everything we do, whether we are aware of it or not, is guided by our system of values. If there is any misalignment between our values and our actions, it will make itself known in how we feel about ourselves and how satisfied we are with our life.

It is also worth noting that some values will get priority over others at different times, and that *prioritizing* values does not mean *going against* our values. Because our values work like an internal compass to help us orient ourselves within the world, they are much deeper than fleeting opinions we may have. When we hold certain values and it becomes our way of living, it gets integrated into who we are *being* and how we carry ourselves. It is our personal work to live and embody our own values, and when we do — it strengthens our sense of Self and sense of Agency. And so it goes without saying that being aware of our values is that much better than to be oblivious to them, because it is the clarity around our values that gives us confidence in our actions.

People often talk about personal values, work values, family values, and so on.

And they talk about them as if these are separate things.

I would like to offer that there is no true distinction. Or, at the very least, we don't need to over complicate things by dividing values into categories like that. The reality is that we bring our personal values into all areas of our lives, be it family, work, or something else.

This happens because values are so essential to what makes us the individuals that we are, that they come with us wherever we go. Just like you bring your eyes and your ears, your heart and your mind wherever you are, you carry your values with you as well. If we don't see our values as consistent across various areas of our lives and if we see some areas as needing a separate set of values that is different from our personal values, then we are more likely to find ourselves in a problematic dichotomy and feel misaligned.

So how do we become aware of our values?

Values are most clearly expressed in the choices we make. Perhaps what you can begin to think about is what values are you currently aware of that guide your actions on a daily basis? Choices you are currently making, big or small, how are you making them and what values do they reflect? This does not need to be something grand, but even just things like tidying up after ourselves, or recycling, or choosing to purchase from one store over another. All of this, when done intentionally, reflects what we find meaningful and important in our lives.

We can also look back at personal dilemma's or difficult life choices to see what drove our decision and whether that decision felt in alignment with ourselves. The choice we make is always in favor of something and that something is what we value. Sometimes these choices are easy to make (when one option clearly goes against our values) and sometimes they are more difficult (when both choices represent our values). For example, deciding whether to eat cake for breakfast, lunch, and dinner, or whether to choose healthy meals instead, is easy when you value healthy nutrition. The cake option is out of the question! However, deciding between working extra hours on the weekend versus spending time with your family may be a very difficult choice, especially when you have a significant financial need but also value quality time with family.

Whereas in the first example the choice is easy because we value one thing over another, the second example is a bit more challenging because both options correspond with our needs and values, which makes the choice harder to make. This is where both values are equally as important, but because a choice has to be made (since you cannot be at work, while simultaneously also having quality time with your family), it will be decided based on what values have priority for you at that moment. So long as we are clear about how and why we are making one choice over another, we can stand behind it, even when they are really tough to make.

When we are faced with difficult choices like that, we may feel guilty for choosing one option over the other. This comes from an underlying assumption and, if you remember our earlier conversation on guilt, someone else's expectation that we should be able to do all things, for all people, at all times. However, there naturally will be times when we will have to prioritize, and some things will move to number one on our priorities list. This does not mean that other things are not valued, but that they will have to wait for their turn. There will also be opportunities to make choices that are in alignment with more than one of our values, which is the best indication that we live in harmony with who we are and what we find important.

When we have a clear understanding of our values, we acquire an internal compass that guides us in the right direction and helps us make the right decisions in life. And when I say "right" what I mean is — the right ones *for you*. That is the whole point. Only when we tune in with *our* values and what is meaningful *to us*, can we find the right direction. That direction does not come from other people's opinions, expectations, or even other people's values. What is right for others may not be right for you. And what is right for you, may not be right for others. It is so freeing to know that, no matter the noise around us and regardless of all the confusion, our values help us tell what is the right thing to do.

Our values also help set the boundaries around ourselves.

They shield what's important from the unwelcomed influences.

Living in accordance with our values and from a place of integrity, frees us from the external pressure of the world, the rules not congruent with us, other people's expectations, conflicting advice and opinions, and so much more. People have the right to give advice or have an opinion, and you, likewise, have the right to not accept it. You do this based on the filter and the boundary of your values. If you don't and you follow others without your own filters and your own sense of direction, you'll waste a lot of time, not to mention — become disconnected from who you are. The personal development industry loves hating filters ("We view the world through too many filters" they say), but the truth is you've got to have them. You need to have them *on purpose* and with intention. It is the "blinders" that help you focus on what matters to you, so that you can make the contribution you are meant to make to your life, your family, and others that matter to you.

Driving from one city to another is a good analogy here. When you are clear on where you are going and you have a reliable navigation system, you don't default to asking strangers on how to get to where you are going or whether you should take a left turn, right turn, or keep going straight ahead. But if you have no idea, then even directions given to you from well-meaning people can be confusing and keep you going in circles. Ever experienced that? Yeah, me too.

Sometimes we do that in life, when we disconnect from our own internal navigation system of values.

Truly understanding what we stand for helps us navigate the plethora of information and advice out there. Values help us filter through the noise and find what we deeply resonate with. Asking ourselves if someone's advice resonates with our values, gives us clarity as to what we decide to do and why. It gives us some much needed confidence to persist and persevere when things don't go our way and when we face challenging times. Not to mention, that when we do ask someone else for help, we know the kind of questions to ask because they arise from what deeply matters to us.

Everyone has opinions on how to live life, how to solve problems, and what is important. Their opinions come from their own perspective, their own needs, and their own values. While the needs are universal and consistent across the globe, their expression — as we have discussed in Chapter 5 — is clearly not. It varies so much from person to person, that it would be silly to assume that we can all make it rigidly consistent and agree on one, and only one, way to live. If someone from another time period or another culture told us we must do such and such precisely per their instructions, like putting a frog into a bucket of milk to prevent it from spoiling (it's a real thing people used to do, by the way, look it up), we would have no trouble turning those suggestions down if they did not resonate with us. We would shrug our shoulders, roll our eyes, maybe even laugh at how ludicrous a particular suggestion may seem to us, but we wouldn't feel guilty about not following it.

The same applies when we hear people's recommendations today.

What they say is guided by their own experiences and values, which may or may not align with ours. We can decline them as something foreign to us and not feel bad about it. To be able to decline the "shoulds," however, we need to know with clarity where we stand and what truly matters to us personally. That is where our values not only serve us to guide us, but also — to protect us from intrusive recommendations and expectations of other people around us.

Our values define the boundaries of our influence on others.

They also define the influence of others on us.

We decide what goes in and what stays out of our territory, the circle of our life. It is OK to have what matters to you protected in a bubble, as it were. Social pressure, whether it's coming from one or many, can make us forget that we have our own zone of wisdom, rooted in our own values. And if that is the case, we can be rest assured that our feelings will rise to let us know that we are not attending to what matters to us.

There are unlimited ways in which society and other people's standards guilt us into things we neither need nor value. You can tell which of the choices you've made in the past were not driven by you but by someone else's opinion. This is often true when we jump on the bandwagon of various social causes without really knowing what they stand for or whether we stand for them. Sometimes we think that other people did their research so we don't have to and we let the group pressure take over our own discernment. But if you think about it, there were also times when, regardless of how many people around you said yes to this or that, you said — no. So clearly, your values on those occasions were so strong that it didn't matter what the mainstream "norm" was.

Whatever helped you stand your ground with confidence then, can also help you going forward.

All we need is clarity around what we stand for and to understand what our values are. That, combined with our attention to our needs, helps us stay within our own zone of wisdom. So it helps to always be asking, why do we do what we do? How are we making our choices? Are we being honest when we say that what we do, we do it in the name of *what truly matters*? The right *why*, the right *reason*, behind the action will guide us towards choices that truly are in alignment with our values.

COMPETING NEEDS

In addition to your values helping you make choices, your priorities should be defined by your *responsibilities*. You are most responsible to those closest to you. You can define "closest" in many different ways, including — based on what matters to you, on what is close to you in your heart. But, when it comes to whom we are responsible for, the one thing we must not forget no matter what, is — ourselves. That is non-negotiable. Our primary responsibility is to ourselves.

- We cannot have values when we do not value ourselves.

The reason why I am bringing this up is that, when we have limited resources or are finding ourselves in challenging times, there inevitably will be competing needs and competing priorities. This means that something will have to come first, at the expense of another thing, which may have to be put at the very bottom of our list of things we want to attend to. And when we are finding ourselves in these times, it is so important to be clear that our choices are driven by our responsibility to ourselves and all that which matters to us.

Stressful times have a way of shaking our confidence overall, which can also make us susceptible to the influence of others. If we are not careful, we may find ourselves making choices based on what other people value, or based on what they told us we should be responsible for. Watch out for that.

The last thing we need to be doing is sorting the tension between other people's needs and the needs of our own. There should never be competing needs that are not ours, since other people are responsible for their needs and we are responsible for our needs. And there is more than plenty to sort out when it comes to our own needs and priorities, because we can most certainly bet that at some point or another, our needs will be in conflict with each other.

The needs of the body may compete with the needs of the Self.

One need of the body may conflict with another.

One need of the Self may conflict with a different need of the Self.

Competing needs are not a problem. We just have to be aware of when it is happening so that we are able to prioritize in a way that works for us. When we choose to attend to something first, it doesn't mean that we consider the rest not important. It simply means that need A is taken care of first, for several reasons, which have nothing to do with importance (as we have discussed, no one need is more important than the other). And as soon as that is met, we move to need B, and so on. How we decide which need to attend to first will depend on several factors, such as our assessment of intensity of the need, our assessment of present and future availability of resources, our subjective sense of what matters to us most in that moment, and, of course, on what we value.

Competing needs can come in unexpected times and look differently depending on our situation. I am reminded of a humorous scene in the movie *Forrest Gump* where he is congratulated by President Kennedy. When asked how he felt, Forrest replied, "I gotta pee." In that scene a physical need takes over a psychological need for acknowledgment. And, by the way, given who Forest Gump is, his need for recognition appears to be better met when people he cares about acknowledge him (e.g., his friends, the love of his life) as opposed to people of high status, even if it is the President.

This is a good illustration of the fact that everything that has to do with our needs — especially when it comes to competing needs — is very individual and personal to our circumstances. Per usual, let me use an example of a physical need, to illustrate this point. Imagine you arrived home late evening after sitting for hours in traffic. You feel sleepy and hungry, you have an excruciating headache, and — why not — you also gotta pee.

Depending on which need is the most pressing for you at that moment, you may first use the bathroom and then take pain medication for your headache before you eat something, and then go to bed. But perhaps, based on your knowledge of yourself, you decide you urgently need something in your stomach before you go pee because you know that, if you don't, you are going to get really nauseous (that's how hungry you are). Perhaps you also know that once you eat, your headache will go away, and so you meet your needs based on that knowledge of yourself. For sleep-deprived new parents, this sequence may look altogether different and, in fact, sleep may be more of a priority for them than food.

Now, I understand that these examples have nothing to do with values. And that makes sense because these are examples of competing *physical* needs. However, the process is similar when it comes to prioritizing *psychological* needs that may be competing with one another. Except here, *our values* become relevant in helping navigate how we meet them and in which order. Say you have very limited time and want to see a close friend but also want to read a philosophy book. What will you do? Which one seems to be more pressing than the other at that moment?

You may choose one thing at one time and another thing at another time, because you still find both of these very important, but at any given moment one value (Relationships or Wisdom) will outweigh the other and be more of a priority.

Choices like these may be tough as it is, and so the last thing we need when faced with tough personal decisions is irrelevant and biased influences of other people, their own judgments and expectations. As we discussed previously, when it comes to our needs, they are always personal to us. What we need is *supposed* to be subjective, because our needs are personal to us. Therefore, we have to rely on our discernment and prioritize based on that. "Is it meeting my needs and/or the needs of those I am *directly* and *reasonably* responsible for?" is a good question that helps tap into our discernment. Choosing out of alignment with what's good for us and what serves us will never make us fulfilled and balanced. Again, we are not talking about being selfish here. We are talking about acting with integrity and being wise with our energy and resources.

- If our own values don't drive our priorities,
  other people's opinions will drive our lives.

That is another reason why having clarity around our values and living in alignment with them frees us from guilt. You see, when we are clear on what we stand for in smaller and bigger ways, then we can have clarity as to whom to listen to, if at all. And so other voices and their judgment become less and less relevant. If we doubt where we stand and allow ourselves to succumb to other people's ideals, we may end up chasing perfection rather than focusing on the most important things for us personally.

When resources are low, it is wise to prioritize in favor of needs, as opposed to the wants. This is something we talked about earlier. It means making sure that before we prioritize one *need* over the other, we actually do our due diligence and prioritize needs over the *wants*. Very often, minimizing or removing certain wants from our list of priorities, helps us see how else and in what other ways we can meet our core needs. We are able to see more resources when we get more clear on what our needs are, as opposed to what our wants may be. This clarity can also come from our values, because it is our values that filter out the noise and help decide how to make choices.

Meeting our needs proactively, which is something we have talked about in the previous chapters, will make us more able to re-allocate resources to meet the demand of shifting priorities so that it doesn't feel like you have too many fires burning all at once. When life is a constant emergency, it can lead to overwhelm (see discussion on burnout in Chapter 7), and overwhelm is the worst place to be when seeking clarity about what is truly important to you.

That is another reason why being proactive in meeting our needs is so important — it reduces the chances of overwhelm. When we meet needs proactively and consistently, there will be fewer conflicts of needs to resolve.

GUILT vs. REMORSE

When it comes to living in integrity with our values and the ongoing necessity to set personal priorities, boundaries is our go-to. Boundaries and their importance cannot be underestimated, and we simply cannot do without them. Guilt plays a huge role in our ability to hold strong boundaries. In order to get hold of guilt and not let it run our lives, it really helps to understand the difference between *guilt* and *remorse*, which may feel similar, but are in fact two very different emotions.

In our society there is no shortage of conversations about guilt and no shortage of opinionated people with big platforms that will tell you what you should feel guilty about. In this context and since it's more common, guilt may feel more familiar as an emotion than the feeling of remorse. However, when it comes to meeting our needs, setting boundaries, and navigating our priorities, guilt is the worst guide and will lead us astray. It has no benefit to us and does not improve our lives in any way. In fact, it results in unnecessary suffering. The good news is that you can learn to let go of it. In order to be able to let it go, you have to see it for what it is and get tired of appeasing it.

Compared to guilt, *remorse* is a very different feeling (even though it may feel very similar to guilt), and it is the one we should pay close attention to. We already talked quite a bit about guilt in Chapters 7 and 8 (see sections "Burnout Beware" and "Resolving Judgment and Guilt" respectively), so in this section we will focus primarily on being able to tell the difference between guilt and remorse, so that you can let go of what does not matter and focus on what does. Knowing this difference is important when it comes to making decisions and understanding what actions are driven by our values, as opposed to by other people's expectations.

As you recall, the feeling of guilt was not included in the three primary emotions we discussed in Chapter 4. Let me remind you why. Guilt, as well as other similar emotions such as embarrassment and shame, are self-referential emotions induced by other people's opinions of us.

When I say "other people" it can be opinions, expectations, and judgments of a specific person you know, but can also be a faceless group of people. For example, judgments we feel from the *society at large* because of societal norms or cultural ideals. And when I say "self-referential" I mean — it is an emotion that references the Self. It speaks to our *sense of Self* — as perceived by others — as opposed to *our needs*, as do all of the basic emotions in the Triad of Discomfort.

Guilt, embarrassment, and shame are, of course, distinct emotions in that they have several subtle qualities that make them different from each other, but the important thing they all have in common is the very reason why they are not included in our discussion of core negative emotions. And that characteristic is that they come from an *external value system*, not our own. And, as such, they can and do misdirect our energy and resources to solving the wrong problem for the wrong reasons. Since guilt and its close cousins are not primary emotions, they do not arise from our needs and, therefore, are not critical to our survival. They are, instead, socially driven (letting someone down, not meeting someone else's standard, etc.), and that is why they can direct our attention away from our needs.

When our actions are guided by other people's standards and opinions, which deep down you do not align with, then following them can lead to appeasing others. Appeasing others disconnects us from ourselves.

If, however, you have standards and values of your own, you will naturally have little concern for what other people think about you and only you will be the judge of your choices. Not only this, but when our values are strong and support our integrity, we become powerful and fair judges of our own actions. And that is where remorse comes in, but more on that in a minute.

If it hasn't become clear yet from everything we have discussed in the book thus far, let me reiterate, that *the only way* we have a complete, grounded, and whole perspective of our Self is through satisfaction of our psychological needs, the needs of the Self. A true, reliable, and stable sense of self-worth and self-esteem does not come from other people's approval and opinions about our worth. It comes from our own ability to see ourselves as worthy and respond to what we need in alignment with our values.

If we lack this self-awareness and, consequently, lack the ability to meet our needs, we will look to other people for approval. And here is where I want you to note that there is an important difference between *feeling Self-Conscious* (which means, seeing oneself from the perspective of the Other and their worldview) and *being Self-Aware* (which means, seeing oneself from the perspective of one's own eyes).

The pursuit of social approval is what makes us self-conscious and susceptible to the feelings of guilt, embarrassment, and shame. Think of it like this. Imagine looking at yourself in the mirror and deciding how you look versus asking other people around you if you look OK. True comfort (and, therefore, confidence) comes from being able to see ourselves with our own eyes and adjust things we need to adjust according to what we see and what we approve of. The moment we turn to other people for approval, we lose the confidence to make that assessment ourselves.

Now let's look at remorse and compare it to guilt.

It has a completely different emotional tone.

When you feel guilt, it is a sense of *someone's judgment* on you. When you feel remorse it is a reflection of your *personal assessment* of what matters to you. Remorse is actually a feeling within the Sadness continuum. And as we previously discussed, all feelings that fall within either Anger, Sadness, and Fear continuums (i.e., the Triad of Discomfort), are personally important to us because they signal about *our* needs.

Contrast that with guilt and you can see that guilt has to do with someone else's values, needs, and expectations. When we fail to meet other people's expectations, we may feel guilt, but if we fail to meet our own needs and our own expectations, what we feel instead is — remorse and disappointment in our own actions.

Guilt comes from feeling *self-conscious*.

Remorse comes from *self-awareness*.

The underlying message that comes with guilt is that, in the eyes of someone else, we are never good enough *and* that we don't deserve something we want for ourselves. Having the feeling of guilt persist over a period of time can add up and create a deep sense of inadequacy — feeling like we are not good enough *no matter what we do* for others (because there will always be someone to judge us and there will always be people who will tell us we are not good enough in their eyes).

This in turn can lead to anxiety and a heavy sense of undue pressure and responsibility, such that attending to ourselves becomes a taboo, which then makes attending to others — a burden. Not good, right?

Guilt is a dysfunctional feeling in a sense that it is not helping us meet our needs. It forces us to prioritize other people's needs, which isn't our responsibility. In contrast to that, the three basic emotions (anger, fear, and sadness) make us aware of our needs and in that sense — they are functional, helpful, and useful. Guilt is not a basic emotion and that is why it offers us no clues about our needs. That makes it dysfunctional and not useful.

When we put attention on other people's expectations, we put attention on meeting *their needs* and make them a priority. Not ours. That is why no matter what we do, when those actions are prompted by guilt, it never feels resolved. Guilt-driven actions do not lead to fulfillment because those actions are not driven by what we need or what we value. Meeting other people's needs does not fulfill our own. We can lie to ourselves, of course, and pretend like doing things from a place of guilt feels natural and serves us, but we would be lying nonetheless.

Now, all of this does not mean, of course, that we do not care about other people or do not want to help them.

What I am talking about is the difference between caring *for* and *about* others vs. caring about what they *think* and trying to appease them just so they think about us differently. It's a futile pursuit that costs us precious resources that could be allocated towards meeting our own needs and the needs of those we are directly responsible for (a distinction we talked about in Chapter 8). And the difference between helping others from a place of our values (for example values like Contribution, Generosity, Service, etc.) as opposed to from a disempowered place of guilt and coercion, is a huge one, with enormous emotional consequences.

What emotional consequences? It is any and all feelings which indicate that you are not attending to what is important *to you*. For example, you may feel Fear because you continue to worry even more about what people think. You may feel Sadness because you continue to neglect yourself, dismissing your needs as non-priorities. And you may feel Anger because deep down you know this is not right and you deserve better. When you understand these emotions and the fact that they point to your needs — the ones neglected while pleasing others — you are better able to refocus. So let's be clear:

Living free of guilt does not make you irresponsible.

Quite the opposite — it makes you responsible for the right things.

If we have a genuine sense of duty, a sense of responsibility, and in our actions fall short of our own expectations and values, that feeling — although at first may be confused with guilt — is actually a healthy feeling of *remorse.* As an emotion on the Sadness continuum, remorse speaks to our own assessment of failure or a sense of loss, such as, a loss of opportunity to do something different instead of what we did. And so it reflects our own system of personal principles, priorities, values, and standards, as opposed to that of other people. In other words, remorse originates from unresolved needs or our own misaligned priorities.

In contrast to guilt, remorse has a softer and quieter energy about it, even though it is a very powerful emotion. It feels more like a deep sense of disappointment in the choices we made, whereas guilt feels like external oppression. Remorse also carries space for self-compassion, whereas guilt does not. The closest I can describe remorse would be like losing a bit of ourselves, a bit of our own integrity when we make choices that are not aligned with our own values. We can always restore the sense of integrity and who we are by moving closer to our values, because that is where our integrity comes from.

Remorse, in contrast to guilt, is a healthy functional emotion, since it points at where we want to be and what to strive for. Guilt, on the other hand, is dysfunctional because all it tells us is that we *supposedly* failed someone else, and yet we are still not feeling compelled to act any differently. That is why you may also feel *resistance* at the same time that you feel guilt. Resistance comes up in response to external pressure, which is what guilt carries with it.

Whereas remorse helps us understand what we feel *compelled to do* differently, guilt tells us what we *should do* differently and yet, if we truly check in with ourselves, we really *don't want to.* And that is why we can feel stuck. Functional feelings help you process things, understand your needs, choose an action, and move forwards. Dysfunctional feelings, on the other hand, keep you stuck and unclear of what serves you.

Remorse *realigns* us with what truly matters, but guilt creates a sense of *conflict* with what matters. Whereas remorse compels us to act to correct things, to be more in alignment with what is right, guilt does not have the same motivating power. This, in and of itself, should also tell you where, naturally, our attention should go.

- When you see this difference between guilt and remorse, guilt will lose its power over you.

The origin of guilt is always *external*, but over the course of our lives, general societal messages get *internalized* as our own "truths." (I put this word in quotes for a reason, more on that in a second.) And when we fail to comply with the "shoulds" dictated by other people, we end up feeling guilty about it, because it *almost feels* like we violated our own standards and our own expectations (which isn't actually the case). And that's the catch.

Guilt makes you believe it is *your* standards and responsibilities you violated, when in fact it is somebody else's. If you truly did violate your own principles and values, then what you would feel would be *remorse* or *disappointment,* not guilt. Guilt always has to do with someone else's standards (perceived or real), not our own. So when you can see that these "truths" are not yours to begin with and these "standards" is not something you aspire to, then you can let go of those expectations and — while you're at it — also let go of the guilt attached to them.

Guilt is usually accompanied by internal dialogue that sounds something like this:

"I feel like I have to, but, if I am really honest, I kind of don't want to and, though I feel bad for not wanting to, I still don't feel like doing it, and so I am stuck..."

Or it may sound like this:

"I should have... even though I don't know how I could have, because it looks like I already did my best, but still.... I really should have..."

And it is this kind of self-talk that makes me want to ask — says who? Says who, that you should have? The answer is usually about somebody else's expectation of us that conflicts with what we want. And if we had a chance to do it over again, it's not at all clear that we would have done something different in the same situation. That is how guilt keeps us in a bind of having made a choice that feels unacceptable by "some" standard (somebody else's) and yet acceptable by another (ours).

Remorse, however, helps us realize that our actions were a genuine misstep and we need to do something different to better align with our own priorities and values. And, in contrast to guilt, if we did have a second chance, we would choose differently. In fact, when driven by remorse and values, we often intentionally seek opportunities to do things differently, to correct that mistake, to adjust course.

Remorse highlights a sense of *personal responsibility.*

Guilt carries a sense of *superimposed obligation.*

Do you sense the difference? We may confuse guilt for the sense of responsibility we have towards other people, and so we may feel obligated to learn to live with this feeling. Yet responsibility is very different from a sense of obligation. A forced sense of obligation makes you feel bound and without a choice, whereas responsibility gives you the power and the authority to act in the way that you decide is right because of your values. There is no sense of agency that comes from guilt and it feels as something that's forced upon you, like punishment. That's why we naturally feel resistance in response to guilt. No wonder why. What is there to do when it is about someone else's rules, or standards, or values? Inherently we would feel like we can't own it and yet at the same we can't let go of it either, because it feels as though it is something we signed up for — to hold the same standard. Did we, though?

The reason why guilt can have such a strong hold on us is that it is always attached to values. Except, not our values, but someone else's.

Where we run into trouble is not differentiating our values from other people's values and, therefore, we can be led by other people's priorities, mistaking them for our own. When values are not being upheld, we get a message about it, and that message comes in the form of a feeling.

The most important part is to be able to tell whether that feeling is guilt (which speaks to other people's unmet values and priorities) or remorse (which speaks to our unmet values and priorities). When it has to do with our failure to uphold our own values, the feeling we feel hits close to home and it is something we acknowledge as our own responsibility. That is remorse. It speaks to our own values, something dear to us personally that we recognize wasn't affirmed.

We feel like we *owe it to ourselves* to do differently, to do better. When we let ourselves down, we feel remorseful for our actions, and we know what to do — we look at our priorities and look at what is important to us. There is always an opportunity to do things better. It is the difference between:

- "*I wish* I had done it differently" (remorse), and

- "*I am expected* to do something else" (guilt)

Remorse helps us reassess our actions and make different choices going forward. Guilt keeps us hostage in a double-bind of supposedly "having to" but not feeling "compelled to." Guilt is superimposed, whereas remorse is very personal. When it comes to our own expectations, we can always sort out what matches better with our values and priorities, whereas it is very hard to keep up with other people's expectations (and that is why it's not our responsibility).

The tricky part is that guilt is so good at masquerading as remorse!

We may need to do a bit of digging to see whether our actions are deeply meaningful to us or whether we feel tied to some external standard we don't truly feel committed to. This is where you will have to do your own thinking.

Each situation is experienced differently because of our personal values. Let's look at some examples to help you see how the same scenario may result in either of these two feelings, and that it all depends on whose standard we are trying to uphold.

An example from earlier in this chapter may be a good one to use to illustrate the difference between what guilt feels and sounds like, as opposed to how remorse does. Let's say you decided to work extra hours over the weekend, instead of spending time with your family. As you work, you are finding yourself wondering whether that was such a good idea after all. If you are feeling guilt, it would be expressed in thoughts such as: "I really should be with my family right now. What kind of partner/parent am I? Who does something like this?" Do you notice how there is an external judgment of you? You are somehow not good enough, don't measure up, failing to meet some external standard of what a "good" parent or partner would do. That's guilt talking.

On the other hand, if the feeling you are feeling is remorse, it will come with a very different set of thoughts. These thoughts will have to do with what you personally value: "Deciding to work extra hours was actually a mistake. I would much rather be with my family right now. I miss them and I know they miss me." Here you see that being with family actually was a bigger priority *for you* and had nothing to do with what someone else might be thinking of you. Given this realization, you may decide to wrap things up sooner, or to make this choice a priority when facing a similar dilemma next time so that you choose in favor of quality family time. You regret the choice you made, which is ok, because sometimes our values are so close to each other and the choices so difficult that it isn't until we decide one way or another, that we are able see how that choice actually makes us feel. It is decisions and choices like this that ultimately help us clarify our values. And that is why values work like a compass. When we are off-course, our values help us see it. Remorse reminds us of that too.

Let's look at another example.

Let's say your current job is no longer satisfying. You know that another position at another company would be a better fit for you. Depending on whose values and priorities float in your mind, you may feel guilty about leaving. If you do feel guilty about leaving, it is because other people's needs, values, and priorities are superimposed as more important than your own. The company you are leaving may need you and, given your role, you know they may have a hard time replacing you. You feel their future burden as your own, which makes you feel guilty. If the feeling of guilt gets in the way of you looking for a better fit for yourself and prevents you from taking a new job, you will end up feeling remorse in the future for not attending to your own needs. If we continue to ignore our needs out of guilt and obligation to others, we will inevitably get resentful.

Here is another work-related example. Let's say you had a confrontation with a coworker. At the end of the day, as you process that interaction, you start feeling something about how that went. If you feel guilt, it is because you may hold an acquired belief that you should always be positive and happy around people you work with. You feel this invisible sense of judgment about how it went. On the other hand, if you feel remorse, that is a sign that you fell short of *your own standards* and wish you could have acted differently. This matters to you because of how you see yourself, as opposed to because you worry about other people's perception of you. You genuinely see where you could do better and you want to do better, because it matters to you to show up more as who you are, in alignment with yourself and your values.

Let's look at a parenting example.

Let's say you got angry and yelled at your child. You will feel remorseful and regretful if, let's say, you value your *relationship* with your child. Maybe your value is *communication* and you let yourself down in how you interacted. You weren't your best, even when you know you can and want to. Because of this remorse and your clear values, you will take steps to repair the situation. You will find opportunities to connect with your child, restore your communication, and strengthen your relationship. On the other hand, if you find yourself feeling guilty in this situation, it is most likely because you think something like "good parents shouldn't yell at their children." At the same time you may feel resistance to this thought because you may feel your reaction was justified, given that your child's behavior did make you angry and was quite upsetting to you.

I hope these examples help you tell the difference between how these two feelings show up for us.

See, everything depends on what *you* hold dear and what *you* prioritize. Not what others tell you (or *have* told you) to hold dear and to prioritize.There is a difference between what *you* consider to be your best self as a colleague or a parent and what is a collective understanding of the "ideal colleague" or "ideal parent." If we are not clear who is in charge of our principles — we or the group — we may end up stuck in a guilt cycle for a long time, forever feeling the dread of never being good enough.

Unless your standards and your expectations for yourself come from you, you will end up feeling guilty every time you fail to meet other people's expectations of you. When we are chasing standards other people set, we will never get it right, because different people have different expectations. That is how guilt ends up stealing our confidence.

The reason why it is so important to be able to tell the difference between guilt and remorse is because, once you can tell them apart, it helps you get unstuck. It helps you to know what to do. As I mentioned earlier, functional feelings (remorse is one of them) help you process things and choose an action that serves you. Dysfunctional feelings (like guilt) keep you stuck and unclear.

So if after some reflection you realize that your feeling is coming from a place of personal values and *you owe it to yourself* to make a different choice given the opportunity (meaning, you realize that what you are feeling is remorse) then you know what to do. What you do — is you make a choice that better aligns with your values.

If however, you discover that the feeling is coming from a place of pressure to do what is "generally" considered a good thing to do and the feeling is guilt, then what do you do? Since guilt is so unproductive and will keep you stuck, you need a way to absolve yourself from it.

I hope reflecting on the following will help you with this.

There are so many expectations and so many voices around us, that it is simply impossible to be everything to everyone. The only thing that makes sense is — to be *your own best*, in alignment with *your own vision* for yourself, who you are, and who you want to be. The only way you can do your best and be your best is to align your choices and actions with your own internal system of values, as opposed to some external standard. In order to do that, it helps to examine your values, to get clear on what you hold dear, and in what ways can you align with what is meaningful to you.

I am an advocate for having only one voice in our head — our own.

That is exactly why we have our own voice, so that we can trust it and rely upon it. We can even ask ourselves again, whether we (without anyone ever knowing or judging us) want or do not want to do something. And if the answer is yes, we can check in with ourselves on whether we want to do it the way we are told to do it. So let's say you don't want to go have drinks after work, who said you should? You really don't have to. If you value connection with your coworkers and would like to spend time with them outside of work, you will find a way to do so, a way that is also aligned with you.

Our own voice can show us whether we agree or disagree with what is being asked of us. If we feel guilty for choosing our own preference, we allow the voice of someone else to speak louder than our own and, by doing that, we are choosing against ourselves. And choosing against ourselves will always result in resentment.

- Anytime you feel the feeling of guilt,
  it is a good reminder to examine your values.

I say this because it is very likely that, if you felt guilt, you are trying to conform to values that are not as dear to you as your own, and that someone got you believing you should really care about. And so, with that in mind, feeling guilt is a perfect opportunity to re-evaluate the standard. Instead of falling prey to presumed sense of obligation and then feeling resentful about it afterwards, take a pause and check in with yourself as to where the feeling of guilt is coming from, and then set your priorities in alignment with *your* values and *your* needs.

This is your own wisdom speaking, so listen to your heart.

It is never wrong.

Final Thoughts & Next Steps

As we conclude this conversation, I hope that you have discovered a different way of looking at your emotions and found a new appreciation for them. Most importantly, I hope that you have experienced a few insights and aha's of your own that make you excited to take your learning further and see the real impact the Needs-Based Emotional Regulation Process (NBER Process) can have on your life.

When applied consistently, this simple 3-step process will allow you to understand yourself and your needs better, which also means that you are more likely to meet them in a way that works for you. Ultimately, this means that more of your needs will be met on a regular basis, and that is the answer to feeling balanced and at peace, and staying within the zone of vitality and aliveness.

We have covered a lot of ground in this book, and you may have questions or want more examples on how to understand needs and find resources to meet them. Since there is only so much that can be said in one book, I invite you to continue this conversation with me and by staying in touch in the following ways:

- Visit my website to access additional resources related to this book. Go to www.dontblamethebrain.com or https://juliapappas.co/dontblamethebrain/. You can also scan the QR code (on the right) with your phone and it will also get you there.

- Listen to my podcast, where I go into more detail on how to understand emotions and apply the Needs-Based Emotional Regulation Process to various needs and situations. Go to https://juliapappas.co/podcast/ or scan the QR code to access the website directly.

- Ask me questions! You can reach out via the contact form on the website at https://juliapappas.co/contact/ or email me directly at info@juliapappas.co

- Work with me directly if you prefer personalized guidance, tailored to your specific situation. Individual coaching can help you understand how this process applies to you and help you access resources unique to you and your circumstances. Feel free to email me at info@juliapappas.co

- Sign-up for email updates, so that you know when I release new resources, books, etc., as well as any supplemental materials that become available related to this book.

- And finally, if you have enjoyed this book, please take a moment to leave a review on amazon.com and tell me what you found to be most helpful. Your input will inform future editions and help me write my next book. And please don't forget to tell others about it!

Appendix A: The Basic Triad of Discomfort

Three fundamental emotions express our discomfort or distress when psychological needs are not met. They are Anger, Sadness, and Fear, as shown on the table. Under each one of them, you will find a list of the more nuanced expressions in the form of other feelings within the same category.

You will notice that these more nuanced feelings vary in their intensity and how much of the basic emotion they contain within them. These feelings are listed in both alphabetical order and also *loosely* organized in order of intensity (*from low to high*).

Moving from low to mild levels of discomfort to high levels of distress, they demonstrate the progression of intensity for that basic emotion, forming a continuum — or emotional range — for that fundamental emotion.

ANGER **& what you might be feeling when you are *angry***		**SADNESS** **& what you might be feeling when you are *sad***		**FEAR** **& what you might be feeling when you are *afraid***	
Alphabetical Order	Order of Intensity	Alphabetical Order	Order of Intensity	Alphabetical Order	Order of Intensity
Annoyed Aggravated Bitterness Defiance Disapproving Exasperated Frustrated Hate Irritated Jealousy Rage Resentment Vengeance	Disapproving Annoyed Irritated ⇩ Frustrated Aggravated Exasperated Bitterness Resentment ⇩ Defiance Jealousy Vengeance Hate Rage	Bored Despair Disappointed Discouraged Grief Hopeless Hurt Lonely Lost Nostalgic Pain Pessimistic Regretful Sorrow Wistful	Bored Wistful Nostalgic Disappointed ⇩ Discouraged Regretful Hurt Pain Loss Lonely Pessimistic ⇩ Sorrow Grief Hopeless Despair	Ambivalent Anxious Cautious Concerned Defensive Dread Insecure Nervous Panic Terrified Timid Worried	Cautious Ambivalent Timid Insecure ⇩ Nervous Concerned Worried Anxious Defensive ⇩ Dread Panic Terrified

MIND/BODY SCAN OVERVIEW

Questions to ask in order to identify which basic emotion is present:

Mind Scan	**If *"YES"***	**Body Scan**
– Does something seem unjust or unfair?	Anger	– Does my body energy feel warm/hot?
– Did/will I lose something? Is something gone?	Sadness	– Does my body energy feel low or heavy?
– Am I concerned something bad will happen?	Fear	– Does my body energy feel antsy, chilled, or cold?

Appendix B: Core Human Needs

This table gives you an overview of basic human needs, which consist of both physical and psychological needs. *Needs are equal and non-hierarchical.* As complex human beings, we must attend to both sets of needs in order to feel balanced, happy, and content. Please refer to Chapter 5 for a detailed discussion.

Needs of the Body (physical needs)	**Needs of the Self (psychological needs)**
❖ Food & Water ❖ Air ❖ Chemical Balance (hormones, nutrients, elements, etc.) ❖ Health ❖ Comfort (absence of physical pain) ❖ Warmth ❖ Rest & Sleep ❖ Movement	❖ Safety & Comfort (Privacy, Stability, etc.) ❖ Agency & Control (Power, Strength, etc.) ❖ Freedom & Autonomy (Independence, Sovereignty, etc.) ❖ Worth & Acknowledgment (Being Seen, To Matter, etc.) ❖ Fun & Enjoyment (Play, Spontaneity, etc.) ❖ Stimulation & Growth (Challenge, Change, etc.) ❖ Intimacy & Connection (Attachment, Belonging, etc.) ❖ Meaning & Purpose (Impact, Contribution, etc.)

Appendix C: Personal Values List

This list of personal values is not perfect, nor is it complete. Its only goal is to give you a sense of what others hold as their values, so that you ponder about your own. It is more important that you ask yourself a question as to what truly matters *to you,* than it is to question the items on this list or to worry as to whether someone else will approve of your values.

Your values are very personal and it is more than alright if you keep them private. Some of your values may not be on this list, and that means you need to add them to it. Return to this list over time and see how your values are shifting and, perhaps, getting more defined and clear.

Please refer to Chapter 10 for a detailed discussion on the role personal values play in our ability to meet our needs and regulate well emotionally.

Abundance
Accountability
Achievement
Adventure
Aliveness
Altruism
Ambition
Appreciation
Assertiveness
Beauty
Bravery
Boldness
Calmness
Candor
Change
Charisma
Clarity
Collaboration
Commitment
Communication
Community
Compassion
Competence
Contribution
Courage
Creativity
Curiosity
Daring
Decisiveness
Dependability
Determination
Development
Dignity
Discipline
Drive
Duty
Education
Empathy
Environment
Excellence
Family
Fairness
Faith
Flexibility
Focus
Friendship
Fulfillment
Generosity
Genuineness
Gratitude
Harmony
Holistic Living
Honesty
Honor
Humility
Humor
Influence
Impact
Independence
Innovation
Intelligence
Integrity
Intuition
Justice
Kindness
Knowledge
Leadership
Learning
Legacy
Logic
Loyalty
Mastery
Moderation
Mindfulness
Nature
Non-conformity
Openness
Optimism
Orderliness
Originality
Partnership
Passion
Patience
Peace
Perspective
Perseverance
Playfulness
Positivity
Power
Privacy
Productivity
Professionalism
Prudence
Purpose
Rationality
Recognition
Respect
Responsibility
Relationships
Reliability
Resilience
Risk-taking
Security
Self-Awareness
Self-Care
Self-Expression
Self-Mastery
Self-Realization
Self-Respect
Service
Simplicity
Solitude
Spirituality
Strength
Success
Talent
Teamwork
Thoughtfulness
Tradition
Truth
Vitality
Vulnerability
Understanding
Uniqueness
Utility
Wealth
Wisdom
Work Ethic
Zest

Appendix D: 3-Step NBER Process Overview

The Needs-Based Emotional Regulation Process (or NBER Process, for short) consists of 3 Steps. The table below gives you an overview of the NBER Process in the form of "What's Wrong?" inquiry, which was discussed in Chapter 3. For more information about each of the steps in the NBER Process, please refer to Chapters 4, 5, and 6.

THE "WHAT'S WRONG?" INQUIRY

Emotional Resonance & Triad of Discomfort	**Need Awareness (Questions We Ask to Find Out)**	**Resource Awareness (Types of Actions to Resolve the Need)**
ANGER	What's not right or fair? What is it that am I trying to protect, fix, or get back?	Actions that restore the sense of justice and make things right.
SADNESS	What didn't work out? What has been lost? What was important?	Actions that honor what is important and preserve what matters.
FEAR	What do I think will happen? What am I concerned about?	Actions that mitigate the threat and provide additional security.
Step 1: "What am I feeling?"	**Step 2: "What am I needing?"**	**Step 3: "What can I do to help myself?"**

You may also find this flowchart to be a helpful reminder of the basic principles behind what we do with emotions when they have a positive (+) or a negative (—) charge. *E* stands for *emotions* and *N* stands for *needs*.

NEEDS-BASED

EMOTIONAL REGULATION FLOWCHART

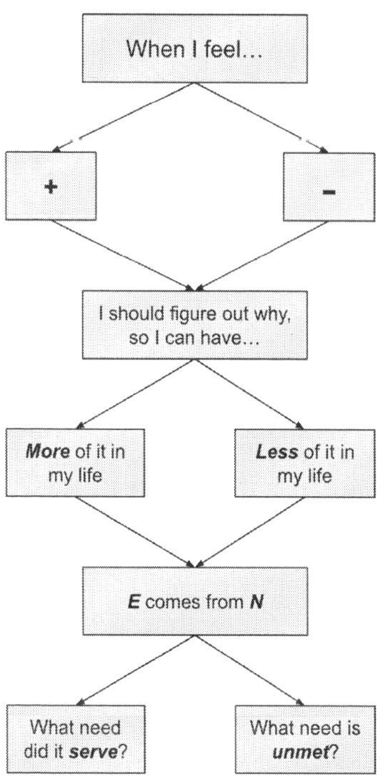

Acknowledgments

What would one do without great friends, peers, and mentors! This book would not be the same without them. Special words of gratitude go to the following individuals for their feedback, support, inspiration, guidance, and mentorship:

Elisabeth Anderson

Julia Anthis

Hisham Beydoun

Laura Carrier

Robin Codding

Lisa Cosgrove

Karen Delano

Theresa Delgado

Angelo DeRosa

Ellen Gillis

Sanaa Kazi

Ilana S. Lehmann

Nancy Modlish

Meghan Mongeau

Angela Oberg

Angie Palaiologou

Konstantinos Petrogiannis

Mukesh Shah

Bethany Smith

Lane Watson

Linda Williamson

*

About the Author

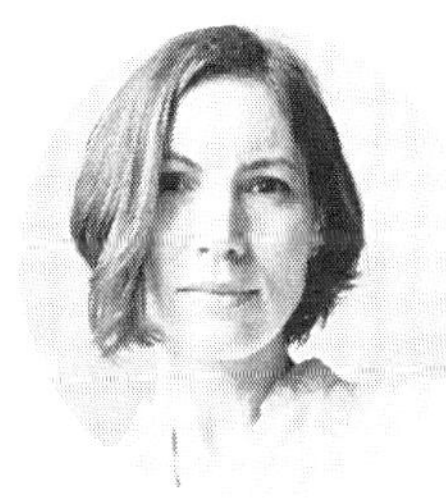

Julia Pappas, M.Ed/CAGS, NCSP, CPC is a Licensed Psychologist, Certified Professional Coach, and Parent Mentor. The focus of her work is emotional regulation of adults and children, as well as improvement in behavioral functioning and mental wellbeing across the life span. Her mission is to make complex behavioral and emotional concepts approachable, by simplifying things down to doable tangible steps. This way, progress becomes not only possible, but also — more visible.

Julia completed her undergraduate degree at the University of Ioannina, Greece and her advanced graduate studies at the University of Massachusetts, Boston, where she also served as a research and teaching assistant. She is the host of The Parenting Presence podcast and a co-host of a local parenting circle. Julia speaks at conferences, schools, and professional organizations on topics of mental health, behavioral and emotional regulation, relational dynamics, as well as parenting.

When not at her desk, Julia makes time for creative pursuits and enjoys being in nature. More about Julia can be found on her website at www.juliapappas.co and on social media (Twitter, Instagram, Facebook) at @juliapappasjoy.

Printed in Great Britain
by Amazon

54597348R00159